Haṭ

(A Treatise on Haṭhayoga)

of

ŚRĪNIVĀSAYOGĪ

Critically Edited
by

Dr. M. L. Gharote
Dr. Parimal Devnath
Dr. Vijay Kant Jha

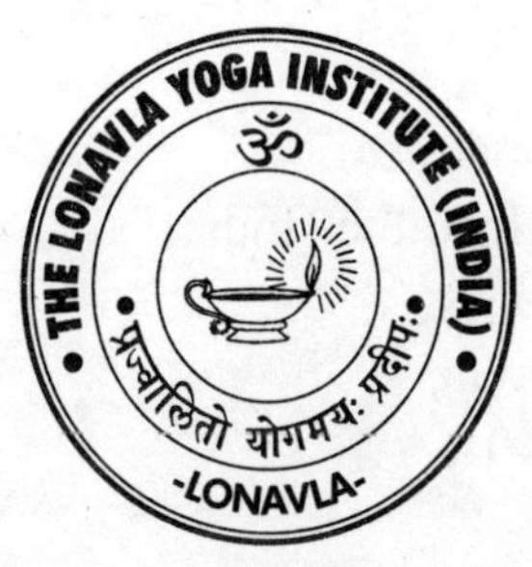

2019
The Lonavla Yoga Institute (India)
Lonavla

First Edition, 2002.
Second Edition, 2009.
Third Reprint, 2014.
Fourth Reprint, 2017.
Fifth Reprint, 2019.

© The Lonavla Yoga Institute (India).

All rights reserved, including those of translation into foreign languages. No part of this book may be reproduced, stored in a retrieval system, or transmitted in any form, or by any means, electronic, mechanical, photocopying, recording, or otherwise without the written permission of the publisher.

Printed by -
Capt. N. Dass (Retd),
XL Images,
S. No. 411/1, Plot No. 11,
Jc. Satish Agarwal Path,
Dapodi, Pune - 411 012.
India.

Published by -
Dr. Manmath M. Gharote,
The Lonavla Yoga Institute (India),
B17, Rachana Gardens,
Bhangarwadi, Lonavla,
Pune. India - 410 401.

ISBN 81-901176-96 Rs. 400/-

Contents

List of Figures

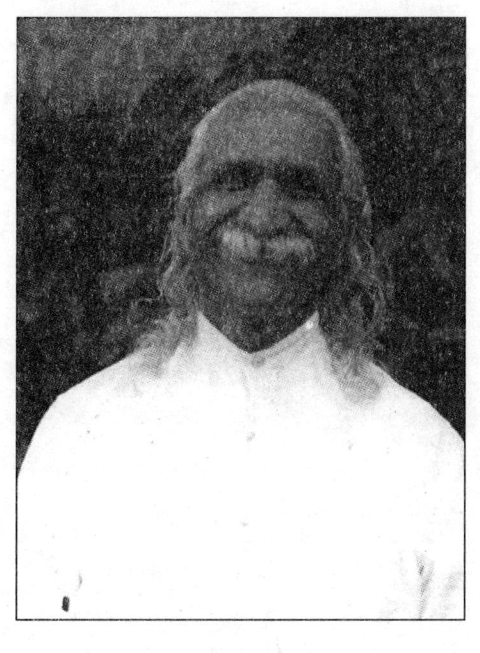

Dedicated

with

profound respect

to

Swāmī Kuvalayānanda

the Source of our Inspiration

for Literary Research in Yoga

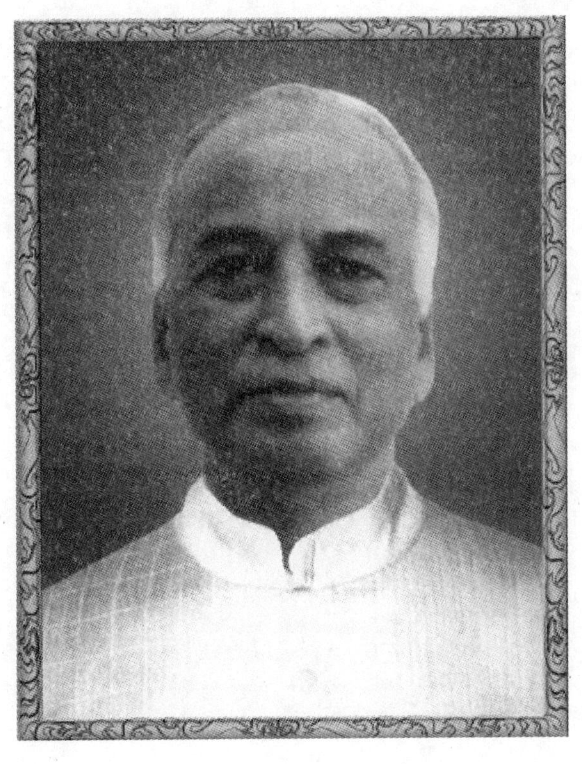

Dr. M. L. Gharote

(21.05.1931—17.01.2005)

एतद्देशप सूतस्य सकाशादग जन्मनः
स्वं स्वं चरित्रं शिक्षेरन् पृथिव्यां सर्वमानवाः

:Manusmṛti-II.20

India has been the land of great masters who lived exemplary life of high moral and ethical order.

Publisher's Note
(First Edition)

We are happy to present our readers this seventh research publication of *Haṭharatnāvalī*, which is an important text of *haṭhayoga* after *Haṭhapradīpikā*.

We feel extremely happy to receive encouraging support and appreciation from the scholars of *yoga* for our research publications so far and we reiterate our promise to publish and present other important titles of *yoga* works to the readers.

We thank our scholars who have been sincerely and enthusiastically working to bring to light important unpublished literature on *yoga*. We hope the readers will appreciate their efforts.

-- *Dr. Manmath M. Gharote*

Publisher's Note
(Second Edition)

I am extremely happy to offer the second edition of *Haṭharatnāvalī* to the hands of Yoga lovers. As other extraordinary publications of The Lonavla Yoga Institute (India), *Haṭharatnāvalī* too has been received by the Yoga fraternity of the world with great enthusiasm. We feel greatly contented to serve the sublime purpose of Yoga.

-- *Dr. Manmath M. Gharote*

Abbreviations

AhS—	*Ahirbudhnya-saṃhitā*
BYS—	*Bṛhadyogasopāna*
DBU—	*Dhyānabindūpaniṣad*
GhS—	*Gheraṇḍasaṃhitā*
GŚ—	*Gorakṣaśataka*
HP—	*Haṭhapradīpikā*
HP (10 chapters)—	*Haṭhapradīpikā,* Lonavla Yoga Institute India)
HP(J)—	*Haṭhapradīpikā* (Ms. No.6756 deposited in RORI, Jodhpur)
HR—	*Haṭharatnāvalī*
HSC—	*Haṭhasaṅketacandrikā* (Ms. No. R 3239 deposited in Madras Govt. Oriental Library).
HY—	*Haṭhayoga*
JP—	*Jogapradīpakā*
JUp—	*Jābāla-darśanopaniṣad*
KP—	*Kumbhaka paddhati*
KKHP—	*Kapālakuraṇṭaka-haṭhābhyāsa-paddhati*
MMPP—	Maharaja Mansingh Pustak Prakash, Jodhpur
MYS—	*Mahākāla-yogaśāstra*
NP—	*Nirañjana purāṇa*

PS—	*Pārada-saṃhitā*
PYS—	*Patañjala yogasūtra*
RORI—	Rajasthan Oriental Research Institute, Jodhpur
RRS—	*Rasaratnasamuccaya*
SKS—	*Satkarma-saṃgraha*
ŚS—	*Śivasaṃhitā*
SSP—	*Siddhasiddhāntapaddhati*
ŚUp—	*Śāṇḍilyopaniṣad*
TBU—	*Triśikhi-brāhmaṇopaniṣad*
TUp—	*Tejobindūpaniṣad*
TVd—	*Tatvavaiśāradī*
VS—	*Vasiṣṭha-saṃhitā*
VU—	*Varāhopaniṣad*
YB—	*Yukta-bhavadeva*
YM—	Yoga Mīmāṃsā
YSC—	*Yoga siddhānta candrikā*
YŚU—	*Yogaśikhopaniṣad*
YV—	*Yogavārtika*

Scheme of Transliteration

Letters, their sounds and description of these sounds

Simple Vowels--

ॐ	om	like	o	in	home
अ	a	,,	a	,,	but
आ	ā	,,	a	,,	far
इ	i	,,	i	,,	pin
ई	ī	,,	ee	,,	feel
उ	u	,,	u	,,	fulsome
ऊ	ū	,,	oo	,,	wool
ऋ	ṛ	,,	r	,,	German

Dipthongs---

ए	e	,,	a	,,	fate
ऐ	ai	,,	ai	,,	aisle (but not drawled out)
ओ	o	,,	o	,,	over
औ	au	,,	ou	,,	ounce (but not drawled out)

Gutturals---

क	k	,,	k	,,	kill
ख	kh	,,	kh	,,	ink-horn
ग	g	,,	g	,,	girl
घ	gh	,,	gh	,,	long-house
ङ	ṅ	,,	n	,,	king or ink

Palatals--

च	c	,,	ca	,,	church
छ	ch	,,	like the sound in Churchill		
ज	j	,,	j	in	join
झ	jh	,,	palatal 'z' in azure		
ञ	ñ	,,	n	in	pinch

Cerebrals--

ट	ṭ	,,	t	,,	tub
ठ	ṭh	,,	th	,,	pot-house
ड	ḍ	,,	dh	,,	dog
ढ	ḍh	,,	dh	,,	mad-house
ण	ṇ	,,	n	,,	splinter or and

Dentals---

त	t	,,	dental 't' as in 'thin' or like the French 'T'		
थ	th	,,	th	in	thunder
द	d	,,	th	,,	then
ध	dh	,,	th	,,	this
न	n	,,	n	,,	no

Labials---

प	p	,,	p	,,	paw
फ	ph	,,	ph	,,	top-heavy or gh in laugh
ब	b	,,	b	,,	balm
भ	bh	,,	bh	,,	hob-house
म	m	,,	m	,,	mat

Semi-vowels--

य	y	,,	y	,,	yawn
र	r	,,	r	,,	rub
ल	l	,,	l	,,	lo
व	v	,,	w	,,	wane

Spirants---

श	ś	,,	r	sh	ashes
ष	ṣ	,,	a strong lingual with rounded lips		
स	s	,,	s	,,	sun

Aspirate---

ह	h	,,	h	h	hum

Nasalised **म्** as in **संयम** (*saṃyama*) --ṃ
visarga--------------------------ḥ

Haṭharatnāvalī

Introduction

Haṭharatnāvalī is an important text of *haṭhayoga* written by *Śrīnivāsa* but not widely known to the students of *yoga*. The author has undoubtedly received the inspiration like many later writers from *Svātmārāma's Haṭhapradīpikā* which occupies a unique position among the texts of *haṭhayoga*.

The text of *Haṭharatnāvalī* was first critically edited and published in 1982 by M. Venkata Reddy who is to be congratulated for bringing this text to light. During the last 20 years after its publication more copies of the manuscripts were available including one commentary in Nepali language. It was considered necessary to edit the text once again on the basis of the available material and improve upon the text by giving transliteration of the Sanskrit text avoiding certain lacunae in the previous edition. For the practical students of *yoga*, it was felt necessary to provide illustrations of the practices, especially of the selected *āsanas*. Some significant readings from the newly acquired manuscripts were also profitably used in this edition.

Materials used for this edition

Eight manuscripts and one printed edition of the text were availed of for collation and noting variations in reading. A brief description of these is given below:

I. Ms. No. 2243 *Haṭharatnāvalī* of *Śrīnivāsa-yogīśvara* containing 4 chapters. Size 24.0 x 12 cm., folios 31, lines 9, letters 24, Nagari script, paper, loose, undated, deposited in the Maharaja Mansimha Pustak Prakash Shodha Kendra, Jodhpur. Indicated as **'J'**.

II. Ms. No. Sa413 *Haṭharatnāvalī* of *Śrīnivāsa-yogīśvara*, size 27.4x13.1 cm., folios 53, lines 12, letters 32-40, Nagari script, Nepali paper, light brown yellow, loose, Vikram Samvat 1919, scribe Cakraman, together with Nepalese translation, deposited in the Rastriya Abhilekhagar, Kathmandu, Nepal. Indicated as '**N**'.

III. Ms. No. 4-39 *Haṭharatnāvalī*, deposited in National Archives, Kathmandu, Nepal, size 38x6 cm., folios 35, lines 4, letters 58, Nagari script, paper, dated Saṃvat 1895, *śrīśaka saṃvatsara* 1760, *śrī* Nepal *saṃvat* 959, *mārgaśīrṣa śukla pañcamī, bṛhaspativāre idaṃ ratnāvalī nāma grantha likhitaṃ saṃpūrṇam.* Indicated as '**n1**'.

IV. Ms. No. 5-6846, *Haṭharatnāvalī,* deposited in the National Archives, Kathmandu, Nepal, size 27.5x6.5, folios 35 (fol. 20th missing), lines 5, letters 32-35, Nagari script, paper, incomplete, undated. Indicated as '**n2**'.

V. Ms. No. 6-1744, National Archives, Kathmandu, Nepal, *Haṭharatnāvalī* + *Śyāmāviṃ-śāṅkākhya yantravidhi*, fol. 20, incomplete, size 29.5x11.5 cm., lines 10-13, letters 40-44, paper, damaged by water, undated. Indicated as '**n3**'.

VI. *Haṭharatnāvalī* in private collection of Yadu Sarma Gorakha, microfilmed by the Nepal-German Manuscript Preservation Project, Reel No. F-30/12, fol. 11, (6-16, 25), incomplete, size 23.5x10 cm., script Nagari, Nepali paper. Indicated as '**n4**'.

VII. *Haṭharatnāvalī* critically edited by M. Venkata Reddy and published by M. Ramakrishna Reddy,

Arthmuru (Andhra Pradesh) in 1982. This edition is based on the Ms. No. 6714 of the MSSM Library, Thanjavur, Ms. No. 5833 from Bikaner Branch of the RORI, Jodhpur. Ms. No. 29860 from Sampurnananda Sanskrit University, Varanasi and Ms. No. 13118-13 of Oriental Institute, Baroda. This last one is incomplete of which nearly half of the text is missing. Indicated as 'P'.

VIII. Ms. No. 6393 (b), *Śrīnivāsena kṛtā Haṭharatnāvalī*, deposited in the Sarasvati Mahal Library, Thanjavur, copied by hand. Indicated as **'T'**.

IX. Ms. No. Re-332-73, *Haṭharatnāvalī* of *Śrīnivāsa*, paper, script Devanagari, pages 1 to 68, obtained from Prof. M. Venkata Reddy. Indicated as **'t1'**.

Prof. M. Venkata Reddy in his Introduction to the critical edition of *Haṭharatnāvalī* has referred to Shri O. Y. Dorasamayya's Commentary of *Haṭhayogapradīpikā* where some *kriyās* like *kilikarma* and *śaṅkhaprakṣālana* from *Haṭharatnāvalī* are mentioned. These *kriyās* are not found described in any of the manuscripts used by us. Similarly, Dorasamayya mentions that he could not find some *āsanas* like *pādapīḍana, nirālambana, vidhūnanam, vicitrakaraṇī, piṇḍamayūra* described in the *Haṭharatnāvalī*.

This indicates that there must be other copies of HR about which we are not aware of. There is a need of locating further copies with different readings of the text.

About the date of composition of HR nothing can definitely be said. However, on the basis of the description of internal and external evidence Prof. Venkata Reddy has tentatively arrived at the period of composition of HR between 1625 to 1695 AD. We also more or less agree to this period of HR.

About the author

Śrīnivāsa, the author of *Haṭharatnāvalī* has given some details about himself in the text. On the basis of this we learn that he was an erudite scholar well versed in the *Vedas, Vedānta, Tantra, Nyāya* and *Yoga.* From his narration, it appears that he wrote commentaries on the works of *Śaśadhara* and *Maṇikānta Miśra.* He also composed the work called *Vedāntaparibhāṣā.*

He was the resident of the Tirabhukta region. His father was a great astrologer, probably named *Saravara* as per the Nepali commentator and the name of his mother was *Somāmbā.* He adores himself with the titles such as *Kalitārkika-cuḍāmaṇī, Sakala-nyāyaśāstra-saṃpradāya-pravartaka, Nyāyācārya, Sakala-haṭhayoga-pravartaka, Jayalakṣmī* and *Mahāyogīndra.*

From the frequent quotations of *Haṭhapradīpikā,* it is clear that he received an inspiration to compose *Haṭharatnāvalī* from *Svātmārāma* although *Śrīnivāsa* criticises him on some points.

Contents of the text

Śrīnivāsa calls his treatise of *haṭhayoga* as *Haṭharatnāvalī.* Alternatively he also calls his work as *Haṭhayogaratnasaraṇī* or *Ratnāvalī.* The contents are divided into four chapters. The distribution of various topics is as follows:

Chapter I

In this chapter after introducing himself, *Śrīnivāsa* gives the purpose of his treatise HR. He gives various definitions of *yoga* and explains *mahāyoga* under which he describes *mantrayoga, layayoga, rājayoga* and *haṭhayoga.* He explains the relationship of *rājayoga* with *haṭhayoga* on the same lines as of HP. He gives elaborate description of eightfold purificatory processes called *aṣṭakarmas* in place of usual *ṣaṭkarmas*, according to the tradition of his *guru*. He criticizes *Svātmārāma* for not including *cakrikarma* under the purificatory processes. He gives a great importance to the practice of *cakrikarma* and recommends it to be practised during *jalabasti* instead of using a tube to be inserted in the rectum for which he also quotes the authority of *yogī carpaṭi*. He provides additional information on the *karmas* like *nauli*, *basti* and *kapālabhrānti* by giving different varieties. Under *nauli* he describes two types, namely, *bāhya nauli* and *antarā*. But the distinction between the two is not clear. *basti* is also described of two types—*jalabasti* and *vāyubasti* for which the use of *cakrikarma* is recommended. In *kapālabhāti* a variety is given wherein the head is moved towards left and right while exhaling rapidly. In the practice of *gajakaraṇī*, instead of plain water, jaggery water or coconut water is recommended.

The purpose of these *karmas* is not only to remove the excess of fat and mucus but to purify six *cakras*, to provide basis for *prāṇāyāma*, to remove all kinds of disorders and to contribute to the healthy body which is an instrument on the path of liberation. It is also described how different *karmas* purify specific *cakras*.

The other topics dealt with in this chapter are description of a hut for *yoga* practice, *mitāhāra*, recommended and prohibited food items, helpful and harmful things in attaining the success in *yoga* and ultimately the list of great *siddhas* who attained success through *haṭhayoga* and conquered death.

Chapter II

This chapter elaborately describes nine *kumbhakas* and ten *mudrās*. Alongwith the eight well-known *kumbhakas*, one more *kumbhaka* is described under the name of *bhujangīkaraṇa. uḍḍiyāna* is called *bāhyoḍḍyāna. vajroli* and *khecarī mudrās* have been dealt with in great detail. The synonyms of *iḍā, piṅgalā* and *suṣumnā* given here are not usually found in other *haṭha* texts.

Chapter III

This is mainly devoted to the elaborate description of 84 *āsanas*. The author starts with the topic of *aṣṭāṅgayoga*, but describes only *mānasa niyamas* and *kāyika niyamas*. No explanation of these is given.

Āsana being the first component of *haṭhayoga* the author deals with this topic elaborately. He gives the list of 84 *āsanas*, but explains the techniques of only 36 *āsanas*. He mentions in the list four types of *padmāsana*, six types of *mayūrāsana*, three types of *kūrmāsana*, and five types of *kukkuṭāsana*. After dealing with the topic of *āsanas*, he discusses the importance, technique and the effects of *prāṇāyāma*.

Chapter IV

It deals with *samādhi* and the techniques like *nādānusandhāna*, four states of progress in *yoga*, such as *ārambha, ghaṭa, paricaya* and the *niṣpatti* and the experiences during each of these states.

There is a discussion of *piṇḍa* and *brahmāṇḍa* in which elaborate description of 14 *nāḍīs* is given as well as philosophical statements from different sources like *Sūtasaṃhitā, Viṣṇupurāṇa, Bhagavadgītā* and different schools of philosophy such as *Nyāya, Prābhākara, Sāṃkhya, Advaita* have been briefly mentioned. This chapter seems to be hurriedly and abruptly ended.

About the Nepali Commentary

Out of the five Nepali manuscripts collected for this critical edition, the 'N' manuscript is all the more important. This manuscript not only contains the text of *Haṭharatnāvalī* but also a commentary on every verse by one *Ambaragīra Yogī.* Who this *yogī* was, is not known. But the scribe *Cakramāna* has copied it in Samvat 1919, i.e. 1862 AD. Except the mention in the beginning about the name of the commentator, no information about his period, his personality, his tradition or his works is available. It seems that he has written a commentary on *Yuktabhavadeva* of *Bhavadeva Miśra*, but we have not been able to go through it. However, it is of great importance for us, since it provided substantial help in preparing this critical edition. *Ambaragira Yogī's* commentary is the only commentary available to us so far. We could not obtain more than one copy of this commentary.

Special Features and Contributions

The characteristic feature of the commentary is its language and style which is clear, lucid and flowing as if he is explaining the contents to a common man.

The explanation about the topics discussed reflects on his experience and rational outlook. Some of the examples are given below.

The term *mahodara* is explained as 'gastric trouble' (i.30). Similarly, while explaining the effects of *neti,* a mention is made about the disturbances in head due to the disturbances of the gastric fire (i.42). In i.44, the explanation regarding filling the stomach with air and pass it out through the anus using *cakrikarma* reflects on his personal experience in the *kriyās* or purificatory processes. Same thing is true also about *basti* on which he comments that after performing the *cakrikarma,* one should contract the *ādhāra cakra.* His mention about the control of fickle mind through the purification of *vāyu* by performing *basti* is certainly valuable (i.52). In the performance of *kapālabhastrī,* suggestion of moving the head to the left and right with the speed of wind denotes a different technique (i.57). In relation to *prāṇāyāma,* the mention of holding the air in the mouth may give surprise to the *yoga* practitioners (ii.43). To attribute *mahāmudrā* to *Vasiṣṭha* is a revelation of new information (ii.41). Invigoration of gastric fire by *jālandhara bandha* may reflect on his own experience. He also suggests adoption of three *bandhas* during *viparītakaraṇī.* These are some of the thoughts exposed by him worth consideration.

Some drawbacks of the Commentary

Despite some of the characteristic points mentioned above, there are many places of errors, which reflect on the ignorance of the commentator. For example, alongwith the mention of 84 *āsanas*, he also mentions 84 *prāṇāyāmas* which do not seem to have any traditional bearing. It is possible that it may be an error of the scribe. While enumerating six *cakras,* the *svādhiṣṭhāna* has not been mentioned. *Brahmacakra* has been mentioned as the sixth *cakra.* These points create perplexity in the minds of the *yoga* readers. He considers *karaṇī* and *viparīta* as separate *mudrās.* In relation to *śakticālana mudrā,* where the reference is made to the length and breadth of the cloth, he considers it the description of *kuṇḍalinī* whose hood is six digits wide and twelve digits long when it is aroused. This seems to be quite irrational. In ii.156, instead of considering the synonyms of *iḍā,* he tried to give the meanings of the terms. There are also errors in the enumeration and description of the names of the *āsanas.* He writes *śilāsana* for *śilpāsana, ardhanāryāsana* and *īśvarāsana* separately *for ardhanārīśvara, śuddhāsana* and *pakṣīsamandrakāsana* separately for *śuddhapakṣī* and *sumandraka.* This creates confusion in the minds of the readers. Although *Śrīnivāsa,* the author enumerates 84 *āsanas,* the number of *āsanaṣ* is much less that is mentioned by the commentator. While describing *vīrāsana,* he strangely calls it *maṇḍukāsana.* In iv.38, he equates *iḍā* with *yamunā* and *piṅgalā* with *gaṅgā,* which is contrary and misleading.

In spite of all these shortcomings, we are thankful to the commentator for the help we derived from it in this critical edition.

A Critical Appraisal of the Text

Haṭhapradīpikā and *Haṭharatnāvalī:* A Comparison

Śrīnivāsa is very well acquainted with HP of *Svātmārāma.* He has quoted the verses from the HP almost verbatim, sometimes acknowledging the source, but many-a-time without mentioning the source. The use of verses from HP in the HR may be mentioned below:

Chapter	no. of verses	percentage
I	23	26.4%
II	53	35.8%
III	43	43.4%
IV	18	28.5%
		134.1 / 33%

Thus it will be found that *Śrīnivāsa* leans very much on the material from HP.

He differs from HP in giving additional information on the following points:

Instead of *ṣaṭkarmas* he describes *aṣṭakarmas*. He includes *cakrikarma* and a variety of *gajakaraṇī* called *gurugajakaraṇī* in the *karmas* or purificatory processes.

HP describes 15 *āsanas*, while HR gives a list of 84 *āsanas* and actually describes 36 *āsanas*.

Although both the texts describe ten *mudrās*, HR has more elaborately described *vajrolī* and *khecarī mudrās*. The mention and description of *saṅketa* is unique in HR because it is not found elsewhere.

The philosophical discussion on the *piṇḍa-brahmāṇḍa* (microcosm and macrocosm) that we find in the HR, is missing in HP.

The synonyms for *kuṇḍalinī, iḍā, piṅgalā* and *suṣumnā* given in the HR is not found in HP.

Contributions of *Śrīnivāsa* in *Haṭharatnāvalī*

In spite of the fact that about one-third portion of the text comes from the HP, there are many special points in this text, which make it an important treatise on *haṭhayoga*. These points are mentioned below.

The concept of *yoga*

The foremost contribution of HR is to remove the misunderstanding about the conceptual definition of *yoga* and to give the clear exposition of *yoga*. The author gives greatest importance to *Patañjali's* definition '*cittavṛttinirodha*' and describes it as *mahāyoga* of which he mentions four kinds, namely, *mantrayoga, layayoga, rājayoga* and *haṭhayoga*. He has defined them adequately as follows:

i. **Mantrayoga**—In the composition of the word *mantra* '*m*' signifies '*manas*' and '*tra*' signifies '*prāṇa*'. The union of '*manas*' (mind) and '*prāṇa*' is necessary in '*mantra*'. When *mantra* is recited after assigning it in the various parts of the body, it is *mantrayoga*.

ii. **Layayoga**—Absorption of mind is *layayoga*, which is attained through '*saṅketa*'. To concentrate at the back of the head at the level of the center of the eyebrows is '*saṅketa*'. Forgetting the objects of experience and absence of their regeneration is the characteristic feature of *laya*.

iii. **Rājayoga**—In *rājayoga, prāṇa* having attracted *apāna* upwards, establishes itself in the lotus of *ākāśa* in the head. In the state of *samādhi*, there are neither the objects of perception nor the activities of the mind. There is an absence of the perception of space and time. One who is established in *rājayoga*, all his awareness is lost.

iv. **Haṭhayoga**-- In *haṭha* the words '*ha*' and '*ṭha*' symbolically represent 'sun' and the 'moon' or '*iḍā*' and '*piṅgalā*' *nāḍīs* and establishing equilibrium between these two is *haṭhayoga*. For this, ten *mudrās*, eight *kriyās, kuṃbhakas* and 84 *āsanas* are the topics discussed in *haṭhayoga*.

In the light of the characteristics of the four *yogas* described above, it could be said that the scope and the content has been clearly presented that is rarely seen in other treatises of *haṭhayoga*.

Aṣṭakarmas

Another characteristic feature of the text is the description of '*aṣṭakarmas*'. Normally a student of *haṭhayoga* is conversant with the '*ṣaṭkarmas*' described in the *haṭha* texts. But *Śrīnivāsa* recognizes '*aṣṭakarmas*' in which *cakri* and *gajakaraṇī* are included. *Śrīnivāsa's* insistence on the practice of *cakrikarma* is so strong that he criticises *Svātmārāma* for having not described it in his HP. He considers the importance of *cakrikarma* in all the *karmas*. He claims that the *cakrikarma* comes from the tradition of his *guru*.

i. Under *aṣṭakarmas*, *nauli* has been described as twofold as *bhārī* and *antarā*. *Śrīnivāsa* has stated that the *bhārī nauli*, which is generally practiced, belongs to *gauḍa* tradition, while *antarā nauli* has been propogated by him. Thus, we find the two traditions in the performance of *nauli*. SKS (114) also talks about *āntra nauli*. However, none of the descriptions is clear to follow the technique.

ii. Another *karma* described is *basti*, which is of two types, *jalabasti* and *vāyubasti*. Although we get their description in GhS also, *Śrīnivāsa* talks about the two traditions in *basti*. One is *Kāpālika* tradition and the other is *Carpaṭa* tradition. In *Kāpālika* tradition, a wooden tube is used for *basti*, while in *Carpaṭa* tradition instead of tube, one resorts to *cakrikarma*. This information is new. *Śrīnivāsa* also gives some useful suggestions regarding the practice of *basti*. For example, he suggests that after *basti*, one should stay in a place protected from draught of wind and should not consume food for about an hour or so.

iii. The technique of *neti-karma* described here is somewhat different from the technique given in the HP and GhS. It not only requires longer thread, but the technique consists of simultaneous friction of both the nostrils, which does not seem to have been described elsewhere.

iv. Under *gajakaraṇī* he gives different technique calling it *gurugajakaraṇī*, in which instead of plain water, coconut water or sweet water mixed with jaggery is used.

v. Commonly known *kapālabhāti* is called *kapālabhastrikā*. *Śrīnivāsa* describes altogether a different technique of *kapālabhastrikā*, not commonly known and practised. It involves moving of the head to the left and right while doing *pūraka* and *recaka*. This movement of head during *kapālabhastrikā* is called *bhrāntibhastrā* in SKS (52). *Śrīnivāsa* attributes the following effects to *kapālabhastrī* : alleviation of the phlegmatic and bilious disorders and diseases caused due to water and cleansing of the forehead and *brahmacakra*.

vi. **Purification of the *cakras*:** In relation with *aṣṭakarmas*, *Śrīnivāsa* has stated how each *karma* brings purification of specific *cakra*. For example, purification of *mūlādhāra* by *cakrikarma*, purification of *svādhiṣṭhāna* by *vajroli karma*, purification of *nābhi cakra* by *nauli*, purification of *anāhata cakra* and *viśuddha cakras* by *dhauti* and purification of *ājñācakra* by *neti* and *trāṭaka*. Similarly *basti* and *kapālabhāti* bring purification of all the *cakras*.

Hopefully, this suggestion of purification of the *cakras* through the practice of various *karmas* may open new vistas of investigation.

Kuṃbhakas

To present traditional facts in a new perspective shows *Śrīnivāsa's* critical outlook. Thus, while describing *kuṃbhakas*, instead of eight accepted *kuṃbhakas*, he includes one more *bhujaṅgakaraṇī kuṃbhaka* and makes the total number of *kuṃbhakas* nine. In this enumeration he omits *plāvinī kuṃbhaka*, but includes *kevala kuṃbhaka*.

Mudrās

While discussing *mudrās*, he provides some new information such as *mahāmudrā* described by *Vasiṣṭha*, practice of *mahāvedha* eight times a day, emphasis on the necessity of a master-disciple relationship for the practice of *vajroli* etc. Detailed description of preparing the tube for *vajroli* practice is also a special feature which we do not come across in other texts. There is quite significant difference about the technique of *śakticālana mudrā*. As against prevalent notion, *Śrīnivāsa* considers *'jihvācālana'* as *'śakticālana'* and calls it *'śabdagarbhācālana'*. Similarly, he gives different synonyms for *suṣumnā, iḍā* and *piṅgalā* which are not seen described elsewhere.

Aṣṭāṅgayoga

It seems that *yama* as a separate *aṅga* under the classification of *aṣṭāṅgayoga* was not acceptable to *Śrīnivāsa*. So he divided *niyama* into two parts and *ahiṃsā* and *brahmacarya* were included under *mānasa niyamas* and *satya* under the *kāyika niyamas*. Thus he does not blindly follow the concepts of ancient tradition on one hand and presents his independent outlook on the other. This independent approach is seen at several places in the text.

Āsanas

In the modern *yogic* perspective, *Śrīnivāsa's* major contribution is in the form of *āsanas*. In many texts of *haṭhayoga*, there is a mention of 84 *āsanas*. But actually they do not give their names and describe only a few *āsanas*. In HR *Śrīnivāsa* not only gives the list of 84 *āsanas* but also describes many of them. Some of these *āsanas* have been mentioned and described for the first time here. The *āsanas* which have been described by him are as follows:

Saṃpuṭita paṅkaja, daṇḍamayūra, pārśvamayūra, padmamayūra, baddhakekī, piṇḍamayūra, ekapādamayūra, bhairavāsana, kāmadahana, pāṇipātrāsana, markaṭāsana, pārśvamatsyendra, baddhamatsyendra, nirālaṃbana, saurāsana, ekapādāsana, phaṇīndrāsana, śayitapaścimatāna, vicitrakaraṇī, vidhūnana, pādapīḍanāsana, vṛścikāsana.

It will not be an exaggeration to say that elaborate description of the *āsanas* is a special feature of HR, which distinguishes itself from the other *haṭha* texts.

Saṅketa

In connection with *layayoga* and *khecarī Śrīnivāsa* has used an important term '*saṅketa*' which needs special explanation. *Saṅketa* means a key through which secret behind any esoteric practices is revealed. In HR, only at two places the word '*saṅketa*' has been used. But *Sundaradeva* has named his treatise as '*Haṭha- saṅketacandrikā*' where right in the beginning he says that to reveal the secrets of *haṭhayoga* the treatise has been named 'HSC'

It has been stated in HR that absorption of mind takes place through '*saṅketa*' and to gaze at *bhrūmadhya* is the highest form of '*saṅketa*'. Importance of the practice of *bhrūmadhya-dṛṣṭi* has been accepted and recommended in all the *haṭha* texts. But *Śrīnivāsa* for the first time revealed the secret of *bhrūmadhya-dṛṣṭi* through *saṅketa*. He has stated that the place of concentration during *bhrūmadhya-dṛṣṭi* is in the back of the head at the level of the center of the eyebrows. It seems that *Śrīnivāsa* considers the place of *citta* here and the concentration at this point may easily lead to the absorption of mind. To explain this point he has used the word *saṅketa*.

Second time he has used the term *saṅketa* in connection with *khecarī*, where the tongue is inserted in the cranial cavity and fixed at the particular place. He has supposed the cranial cavity as zigzag, spiral and consisting of the two chains of *iḍā* and *piṅgalā*. He explains *saṅketa* as inserting the tongue in the spiral of these two chains which reaches the place of *suṣumnā* resulting in absorption of the nectar oozing out of the moon situated there. Students of *yoga* very well know that *citta, khecarī mudrā, candra* are such esoteric terms which are not clearly explained and there is much ambiguity about them. *Śrīnivāsa* has made an attempt to throw some light on these secrets. Therefore, his attempt is very valuable in the field of *yoga*.

For the fear of inflation of the text although elaborate discussion of all the topics could not be attempted by the author, yet there are some new topics like *piṇḍa-brahmāṇḍa-nirūpaṇa, pañcīkaraṇa,* number of *tattvas,* which seem essential for the students of spiritual culture, which have been included in the fourth chapter.

In the light of the above discussion, it can be unhesitatingly said that boldly refuting the prevalent ideas and introduction of new thoughts in a lucid manner, gives a special place to HR among the texts of *haṭhayoga*.

Therapeutical Effects of *haṭhayogic* Practices

Śrīnivāsa has attributed certain therapeutical effects to the various *yogic* practices which are mentioned below:

Name of the practices	Therapeutical benefits
aṣṭakarmas	Effective in cleansing the body, removes the impurities such as fat and phlegm contributing physical well-being.
cakri-karma	Removes piles, diseases of spleen, abdominal disorders, cleanses the morbidities, stimulates gastric fire, purifies perineal region.
nauli	Stimulates gastric fire, improves digestion, feeling of well-being, removes the disorders of the three humours.
dhauti	Removes the diseases like cough, asthma, spleen disorders, skin diseases, all the twenty varieties of phlegmatic disorders.
neti	Cleanses the frontal sinuses, offers keen eyesight, removes the diseases above the neck.
basti	Removes spleen disorders, abdominal disorders, disorders caused by the three humours.
jalabasti	Streamlines the bodily constituents, brings about poise to the sense organs, offers lustre to the body, stimulates digestive fire, alleviates the chronic disorders.
gajakaraṇī	Cleanses the whole tract from stomach to the throat.
trāṭaka	Removes eye-disorders and drowsiness.
kapālabhastrikā	Alleviates the phlegmatic and bilious disorders and diseases caused due to water, cleanses the forehead and *brahmacakra*.

Name of the practices	Therapeutical benefits
vajrolī karma	Cleanses the generative organ.
prāṇāyāma	Purification of the *nāḍīs*, alleviates all the diseases.
sūryabhedana	Removes lethargy, rheumatism and worms.
ujjāyī	Cures the phlegmatic disorders of the throat, increases the bodily fire, removes the morbidities of the *nāḍīs*, stomach and the bodily constituents.
sītkāra	One becomes like a cupid, does not suffer from hunger, thirst, sleep and drowsiness.
śītalī	Removes dropsy, disorders of the spleen, fever, acidity, toxicity, controls hunger and thirst.
bhastrikā	Cures the disorders due to vitiation of *vāta*, *pitta* and *kapha* humours, stimulates the gastric fire.
mahāmudrā	Ailments like consumption, skin-diseases, constipation, glandular enlargement, indigestion are cured. Removes old age and fear from death.
mahābandha	Promotes the currents of the *nāḍīs* moving in the upward direction, fixes the mind between the eyebrows.
mahāvedha	Destroys multitude of sins, alleviates old age and fear from death.
uḍḍiyānabandha	Complexion.
mūlabandha	*Apāna* and *prāṇa vāyus* get unified, urine and faeces are reduced.

Name of the practices	Therapeutical benefits
jālandharabandha	Removes old age and premature death.
viparītakaraṇī	Stimulates gastric fire, alleviates all the disorders, removes grey hair and wrinkles.
vajrolī	Unifies *apāna* and *prāṇa,* cleanses the *nāḍīs*, makes the genital strong, stable and offers increment of semen. Awakens *kuṇḍalinī.*
śakticālana	Removal of diseases.
khecarī	One remains unaffected by diseases, sleep, hunger, thirst, stupor, poison and death.
āsanas	Contributes to stability, health and efficient body. Contributes to a sense of well-being.
bhadrāsana	Removes all the diseases and toxins.
padmāsana	Alleviates all the diseases.
mayūrāsana	Removes diseases of the spleen, stomach, balances the three humours in the body, digests excess food, stimulates gastric fire.
pīṇḍamayūra	Cures all the ailments.
maṇḍūkāsana	Removes the diseases of the legs.
matsyendrāsana	Enhances the gastric fire, removes severe diseases, brings stability to the spine.
phaṇīndrāsana	Removes all the ailments.
paścimatāna	Stimulates gastric fire, reduces the belly, brings good health.
śavāsana	Relieves fatigue.
nādānusandhāna	Contributes to steadiness of the mind.

Śrīnivāsa's Shortcomings

Notwithstanding special contributions of *Śrīnivāsa* described above there are some places which reflect on the shortcomings of *Śrīnivāsa.* They may be stated below:

The author reflects on his egotistic personality when he egotises his scholarly background and talks about his versatility in *Veda, Vedānta,* grammar, philosophy, *tantra,* astrology, etc. At the end of the first chapter, he claims to be a great promoter of *haṭhayoga.*

He unnecessarily critcises *Svātmārāma* for not describing the *cakrikarma* calling it as his ignorance about *haṭhakriyās.*

Although *Śrīnivāsa* talks about the two types of *nauli,* the description of *antarā* type does not differentiate its technique from that of *bhārī* or *bāhya* type of *nauli.*

He says that *svādhiṣṭhāna cakra* is purified by *vajrolī karma,* but does not describe the process.

Similarly, he adds *bhujaṅgakaraṇī kuṃbhaka* in the list of *kuṃbhakas,* but the description is not clear.

He gives great importance to *śāṃbhavī-mudrā* (iv.27). But he describes neither in the description of *mudrās,* nor elsewhere he to it.

In the beginning of the 3rd chapter *Śrīnivāsa* undertakes to describe *aṣṭāṅga-yoga.* But he does not discuss any thing about *yama, pratyāhāra, dhāraṇā, dhyāna* which are included under *aṣṭāṅgayoga.* He mentions *niyamas* and divides them into *kāyika* (physical) and *mānasika* (mental). There is no justification given for this classification. He does not also feel the need of explaining them. Curiously enough, *ṛta* and *satya* are included under *kāyika-niyamas* and *ahiṃsā* and *brahmacarya* are included under the *mānasa-niyamas.*

While considering *aṣṭāṅgayoga,* he talks about *āsana* as the first component of *haṭhayoga* and further elaborately deals with the 84 *āsanas.* This reflects not only on the propriety but also on absence of the coordination in the topics of presentation.

Śrīnivāsa gives the list of 84 *āsanas* but describes only 34 *āsanas.* There too he changes the names of some *āsanas* while describing them. So there is a disparity between the names of *āsanas* mentioned in the list and the names mentioned in the description. For example, instead of *bandhamayūra,* he uses the name *baddhakekī.* Similarly, for *kārmuka* he uses *dhanurāsana.* He describes *saurāsana,* but it is not included in the list of 84 *āsanas.*

In chapter iii.77, he mentions the effects of *pratyāhāra* as destroying mental disturbances but nowhere he explains the term *pratyāhāra.* Same thing is true about *samādhi* (iv.3). He frequently says that due to the fear of expansion of the text, all the details are not described. Such statements do not satisfy the inquisitiveness of the readers.

Even the fourth concluding chapter seems to have hurriedly finished. Since *Śrīnivāsa* claims himself to be the scholar of so many sciences *(śāstras),* readers expect some illumination on such philosophical topics like *piṇḍa-brahmāṇḍa-nirṇaya, pañcīkaraṇa, tatvas* and different traditions and schools of philosophy. But they are disappointed due to the lack of elaboration and explanations.

Plan of Presentation

The original *Saṃskṛta* verse is given first followed by the transliteration in Roman characters. Then against the number of verses is given the translation in English. After this is given against the same number critical note on the topic wherever it was found necessary. Variant readings are given in the footnotes.

In the Appendix-1 are given the extra lines appearing in the Tanjavur ms. No.6393(b) in the chapter iv. Appendix-2 gives the variations of the names of *siddhas* found in different manuscripts of HR and HP. Appendix-3 gives some of the *āsanas* mentioned in the list but not described in the text are described here from other sources.

The important terms have been explained in the Glossary. The index of half-verses gives at a glance all of the verses alphabetically arranged. The index of the words will facilitate the readers to locate information related to the word or topic.

Grateful acknowledgements are extended to the following:

Prof. M. Venkata Reddy for providing a copy of the manuscript and a paper on the text. Dr. Mahesh Raj Pant and Dr. Catherina Kienlhe for arranging to supply the photocopies of the manuscripts deposited in the National Archives, Kathmandu, Nepal; Director, Maharaja Mansimha Pustak Prakash, Jodhpur, for the supply of photocopy of the manuscript deposited with them; Director, Sarasvati Mahal Library, Tanjavur.

We also thank our friends who helped us in the project but prefer to remain anonymous.

Dr. M. L. Gharote
Dr. Parimal Devnath
Dr. Vijay Kant Jha

हठरत्नावली

प्रथमोपदेशः

श्रीगणेशाय नमः[1]

Śrī-gaṇeśāya namaḥ !

Tr. Salutation to *Śrī-gaṇeśa* !

[2]श्रीआदिनाथं नत्वाऽथ श्रीनिवासो महामतिः ॥
हठरत्नावलीं[3] धत्ते योगिनां कण्ठभूषिताम्[4] ॥ 1 ॥

śrī-ādināthaṃ natvā'tha śrīnivāso mahāmatiḥ ॥
haṭharatnāvalīṃ dhatte yogināṃ kaṇṭhabhūṣitām ॥ 1 ॥

Tr. After saluting *Śrī-ādinātha*, the great scholar *Śrīnivāsa* composes *Haṭharatnāvalī*, which adorns the neck of the *yogīs*.1.

वेदे[5] वेदान्तशास्त्रे फणिपतिरचिते शब्दशास्त्रे स्वशास्त्रे
तन्त्रे प्राभाकरीये कणभुगभिहिते[6] न्यायरत्नार्णवेन्दुः[7] ॥
सांख्ये सारस्वतीये विविधमतिमते[8] तत्वचिन्तामणिज्ञः
श्रीमज्ज्योतिर्विदग्रे सरवर[9]तनुजो राजते श्रीनिवासः ॥ 2 ॥

vede vedāntaśāstre phaṇipatiracite śabdaśāstre svaśāstre
tantre prābhākarīye kaṇabhugabhihite nyāyaratnārṇavenduḥ //
sāṃkhye sārasvatīye vividhamatimate tattvacintāmaṇijñaḥ
śrīmajjyotirvidagre saravaratanujo rājate śrīnivāsaḥ // 2 //

Tr. The son of *Saravara*, the great astrologer, *Śrīnivāsa* is a scholar of the *Veda, Vedānta, Pātañjala Yoga, Grammar, Yoga, Tantra, Prābhākarīya, Vaiśeṣika* (of *Kaṇāda*), *Nyāyaratna*, (of *Maṇikānta Miśra*), *Sāṃkhya, Sārasvatīya, Vaiśeṣika* and *Tatvacintāmaṇi* (of *Gaṅgeśa Upādhyāya*). 2.

Note : ***Veda***— The primary scriptures of Hindus are revered as "of divine origin". *Vedas* are four in number, named as *Ṛgveda, Yajurveda, Sāmaveda* and *Atharvaveda*. *Vedas* consist primarily of four collections, which are generally classified as *Saṃhitā*,

---

1. श्री रामब्रह्मणे नमः-P,T,t1, श्रीगणेशाय नमः-n1,n2. 2. ॐ अधिकः पाठः-P,T,t1. 3. हठरत्नावलिं-P,n1. 4. कर्णभूषिताम्-T,t1. 5. वेद–T. 6. शशधररचिते-P,T,t1, विविधश्रुतिमते-J,N,n1,n2. 7. न्यायरत्नार्णवेन्दौ-P. 8. कणभुगभिहिते-P,T,t1. 9. श्रीमज्ज्योतिर्विदग्रेश्वर–P, ज्योतिर्विदग्रेसरवर-J,N,-सरवर-n1,t1.

Brāhmaṇa, Āraṇyaka and *Upaniṣad. Vedas* were not written but 'heard' and transferred to the next generation by oral method.

Vedānta — It is one of the six orthodox systems of Indian philosophy, founded on the *Upaniṣads.* It is also called '*Uttara Mīmāṃsā*'. It was first formulated by *Bādarāyaṇa* in the form of *Brahma-sūtra*, also called *Vedāntasūtra. Vedānta* is uncompromisingly monistic. *Śaṅkara's* interpretation and exposition is regarded as the culmination of the *Vedānta* system. He turned the *Vedānta* into the strictest form of monism.

Phaṇipati — A synonym for *Patañjali*, who in tradition is considered as an incarnation of lord of the serpents.

Śabdaśāstra — It refers to the grammar, particularly, a commentary by *Patañjali* on the *Saṃskṛta* grammar of *Pāṇini.*

Svaśāstra — Refers to *Yoga-śāstra* of *Patañjali.* Nepali commentator *Ambargira Yogī* reads this as *svaraśāstra* which means science of *svaras.*

Śaśadhara — A famous author of *Nyāya-siddhānta-dīpa* on which *Śrīnivāsa* wrote a commentary.

Tantra — The canon of Tantrism is called *Tantra,* which is believed to have been revealed by *Śiva* as the specific scripture for the present times. A large part of the *Tantra* scriptures is written in the form of a dialogue between *Śiva* and his consort *Pārvatī.* Conventionally the topics treated by the *Tantras* are: i) creation of the universe (*sṛṣṭi*), ii) its dissolution (*pralaya*), iii) worship of the deities, iv) spiritual practices (*sādhanā*), v) rituals, vi) supernatural powers (*siddhis*), vii) meditation (*dhyāna*). The literature of *tantras* is abundant and was composed from 7th century to 17th century and is still untranslated. Much of the literature is couched in crude form of *Saṃskṛta* and more often using double entendres which makes the meaning difficult to understand.

Prābhākarīya — It is a school of the *Mīmāṃsā* system of philosophy founded by *Prabhākara.* It admits five different sources of knowledge, namely, perception (*pratyakṣa*), inference (*anumāna*), comparison (*upamāna*), testimony (*śabda*) and postulation (*arthāpatti*). The first four are admitted as in the *Nyāya* system. According to this school, knowledge arises by postulation (*arthāpatti*) also. Although it believes in the reality of the souls, it does not believe in the supreme soul or God. It admits the law of *karma* as a spontaneous moral law that rules the world. Therefore, any ritual performed by man creates a potency in his soul, which produces the fruit of the action at an appropriate time in future.

Kaṇabhug— A system of *Kaṇāda* known as *Vaiśeṣika. Kaṇāda* is also known as *Ulūka.* It is allied to *Nyāya* system of philosophy. It divides all objects of knowledge under the seven categories, namely, substance (*dravya*), quality (*guṇa*), action (*karma*), generality (*sāmānya*), particularity (*viśeṣa*), the relation of inherence (*samavāya*) and nonexistence (*abhāva*). With regard to God and the liberation of the individual soul, the *Vaiśeṣika* theory is substantially the same as that of *Nyāya.*

Nyāyaratna— *Maṇikānta* is the author of an important text on *Navya-nyāya* entitled '*Nyāya-ratna*'.

Sāṃkhya—An ancient system of Indian philosophy of dualistic realism, attributed to the sage *Kapila.* It admits two ultimate realities, *Puruṣa* and *Prakṛti,* which are independent of each other. *Puruṣa* is the power of consciousness, while *Prakṛti* is material cause of the world. *Prakṛti* consists of three *guṇas,* namely, *satva, rajas* and *tamas.* The evolution of the world starts by the association of the *Puruṣa* with *Prakṛti* which disturbs the original equilibrium of *Prakṛti* and it moves to action. In the course of evolution 24 principles are evolved including *Prakṛti*. *Sāṃkhya* does not admit the existence of God. *Puruṣa*, according to it, is neither the cause nor the effect of anything.

Sārasvatīya—Well-versed in the grammar composed by *Anubhūtisvarūpācārya*.

Tatvacintāmaṇi— An important text written by *Gaṅgeśa Upādhyāya* of 14th century.

Saravara— The Nepali commentator *Ambargira Yogī* considers *Saravara* as the name of the father of *Śrīnivāsa*. 2.

हठविद्यां हि[1] गोरक्षमत्स्येन्द्राद्या[2] विजानते ॥
आत्मारामोऽपि जानीते श्रीनिवासस्तथा स्वयम् ॥ 3 ॥

haṭhavidyāṃ hi gorakṣamatsyendrādyā vijānate //
ātmārāmo'pi jānīte śrīnivāsastathā svayam // 3 //

Tr. *Gorakṣa, Matsyendra* and *Ātmārāma* know the science of *haṭha*. So also *Śrīnivāsa* himself. 3.

Note: *Gorakṣanātha*— He was a *yogī* par excellence, famous religious leader, reformer and leading exponent of *Nāthapantha*. There is a mass of literature associated with his name. 10th century has been considered the date of *Gorakṣanātha*. SSP and GŚ are important texts on his name.

Matsyendra— He probably flourished in 5th or 6th century AD. He is regarded as the disciple of *Ādinātha*. He taught *yoga* to *Gorakṣanātha* in 10th century AD. The text called *Matsyendrasaṃhitā* ascribed to him states that he was a fisherman who lived on an island surrounded by the sea and rivers and often used to go on fishing expedition. *Abhinavagupta* mentions him to be the originator of *Kaula* tradition preceding him by 18 generations. The following works are ascribed to *Matsyendranātha*:

---

1. हि – अनुपलब्धः -n1. 2. मत्स्येन्द्रगोरक्षाद्या-P,T,t1.

1. *Kaulajñānanirṇaya,*
2. *Akulavīratantra,*
3. *Kulārṇavatantra,*
4. *Jñānakārikā,*
5. *Kāmākhyāguhyasiddhi,*
6. *Matsyendrasaṃhitā.*

In *Śābaratantra*, he is described as one of the 12 *Kāpālika gurus* renowned for *yoga.* He is accorded the first place in the list of Tibetan *siddhas.*

Ātmārāma — A synonym used for *Svātmārāma.* We find the name *Ātmārāma* used in several MSS of HP instead of *Svātmārāma. Bālakṛṣṇa*, a commentator of HP (10 chapters), uses the name *Rāmanātha* for *Svātmārāma.* 3.

भ्रान्त्या बहुमतध्वान्ते[1] राजयोगमजानताम्[2] ||
केवलं राजयोगाय हठविद्योपदिश्यते || 4 ||

bhrāntyā bahumatadhvānte rājayogamajānatām //
kevalaṃ rājayogāya haṭhavidyopadiśyate // 4 //

Tr. The science of *haṭhayoga* is being imparted only to explain *rājayoga* to those who are perplexed by the varied opinions and are ignorant of *rājayoga.* 4.

अथातो योगजिज्ञासा[3] शास्त्रमाद्यमिदं कृतम् ||
योगस्य विषयं वक्तुं योगशास्त्रे[4] प्रयोजनम् || 5 ||

athāto yogajijñāsā śāstramādyamidaṃ kṛtam //
yogasya viṣayaṃ vaktuṃ yogaśāstre prayojanam // 5 //

---

1 . बहुमतध्वान्तै-J,N,n1.2 . राजमार्गमजानतः-P,T,t1. 3 . योगविज्ञासा-N .
4 . योगशास्त्र-J,N,n1,n2.

Tr. With the desire of knowing traditional *yoga* this foremost treatise has been written. The purpose of this treatise of *yoga* is to explain the contents of *yoga*. 5.

Note: The expression "*athāto yoga-jijñāsā*" seems to have been used on the lines common to the opening verse or line of different philosophical systems in which *Śrīnivāsa* was well-versed. This expression seems to be an influence similar to the one expressed in the texts studied by him. 5.

अपान[1]प्राणयोश्चापि जीवात्मपरमात्मनोः[2] ||
योगश्चायं हि[3] योगार्थं केचिदाचक्षते बुधाः[4] || 6 ||

apānaprāṇayoścāpi jīvātmaparamātmanoḥ //
yogaścāyaṃ hi yogārthaṃ kecidācakṣate budhāḥ // 6 //

Tr. Some scholars opine that *yoga* is the union of *apāna* and *prāṇa,* while others say that it is the union of *jīvātmā* and *Paramātmā.* Yet according to some, *yoga* is for the sake of *yoga* itself.6.

चित्तवृत्तिनिरोधस्तु महायोगः प्रकीर्तितः ||
योगश्चतुर्विधः प्रोक्तो योगज्ञैः सर्वसिद्धिदः || 7 ||
cittavṛttinirodhastu mahāyogaḥ prakīrtitaḥ //
yogaścaturvidhaḥ prokto yogajñaiḥ sarvasiddhidaḥ // 7 //

Tr. Control of the mental fluctuations is called *mahāyoga.* The adepts of *yoga* classify this (*mahā*) *yoga* into four types, which bring about all the *siddhis* (supernatural powers).7.

Note: In these verses, the author tries to give definition of *yoga* in different traditions. *Cittavṛttinirodha* is the definition given by *Patañjali* (PYS-i.2). 6-7.

मन्त्रयोगो लयश्चैव राजयोगस्तृतीयकः ||
हठयोगश्चतुर्थः स्यात् प्राणिनां मोक्षदायकः[5] || 8 ||

---

1 . अपाण-N,n1. 2 . जीवात्मपरमात्मनो- N.3.हि-अनुपलब्धपाठः-n1. 4 . वुधाः-N. 5 . मोक्षसाधकः-P,T,t1.

mantrayogo layaścaiva rājayogastṛtīyakaḥ //
haṭhayogaścaturthaḥ syāt prāṇinām mokṣadāyakaḥ / 8 /

Tr. The four types of *yoga* are – *mantrayoga, laya, rājayoga* the third and *haṭha-yoga* the fourth, which offer salvation to the living beings. 8.

Note: The fourfold *yoga* is designated as *mahāyoga*, which consists of *mantrayoga, layayoga, rājayoga* and *haṭhayoga*. However, the sequence given here differs from the other traditions in which *mahāyoga* is described as follows in YŚU- i.129:

मन्त्रो लयो हठो राजयोगान्ता भूमिकाः क्रमात् ॥
एक एव चतुर्द्धायं महायोगोऽभिधीयते ॥

mantro layo haṭho rājayogāntā bhūmikāḥ kramāt //
eka eva caturddhā'yaṃ mahāyogo'bhidhīyate //

(*Mantra, laya, haṭha* and *rājayoga* in this sequence, are fourfold *yoga* known as *mahāyoga*). 8.

अथ मन्त्रयोगः[1] –
अंगेषु मन्त्रं विन्यस्य[2] पूर्वमन्त्रं[3] जपन् सुधीः ॥
येन केनापि सिद्धः स्यात् मन्त्रयोगः स उच्यते ॥ 9 ॥

atha mantrayogaḥ –
aṅgeṣu mantraṃ vinyasya pūrvamantraṃ japan sudhīḥ /
yenakenāpi siddhaḥ syāt mantrayogaḥ sa ucyate // 9 //

Tr. The wise should recite a *mantra* after assigning it on the limbs. Thus all can attain success. This is called *mantra-yoga*. 9.

Note: It has been emphasized that in *mantrayoga* it is not only the repetition of *mantra* but also placing different parts of *mantra* in the form of *nyāsa* in different regions of the body. 9.

अथ लययोगः –
लययोगश्चित्तलयात्[1] संकेतैस्तु प्रजायते ॥

---

1. अनुपलब्ध –N,n1,n2. 2. मन्त्रमभ्यस्य-P,t1. 3. पूर्वमंत्र-N,T.

आदिनाथेन तु लयाः[2] सार्द्धकोटिरुदीरिताः[3] || 10 ||

atha layayogaḥ —

layayogaścittalayāt saṅketaistu prajāyate //

ādināthena tu layāḥ sārddhakoṭirudīritāḥ // 10 //

Tr. Absorption of mind is *layayoga* which is attained through *saṅketa*. This is *layayoga*. *Ādinātha* has propagated one and half-crore variations of *laya*. 10.

भ्रूमध्ये दृष्टिमात्रेण परः संकेत उच्यते ||
शिरः[4]पाश्चात्यभागस्य ध्याने मृत्युञ्जयः परः || 11 ||

bhrūmadhye dṛṣṭimātreṇa paraḥ saṃketa ucyate //

śiraḥ pāścātyabhāgasya dhyāne mṛtyuñjayaḥ paraḥ // 11 //

Tr. Fixing of the gaze at the center of the eyebrows is the finest *saṃketa*. By concentrating at the rear side of the head, one overcomes death. 11.

एतदेव[5] मतं सम्मतं[6] हठप्रदीपिकायामपि –

श्रीआदिनाथेन सपादकोटिलयप्रकाराः कथिता जयन्तु ||
नादानुसन्धानकमेव कार्यं[7] मन्यामहे मान्यतमं लयानाम् || 12 ||

etadeva matam sammatam haṭhapradīpikāyāmapi —

śrīādināthena sapādakoṭilayaprakārāḥ kathitā jayantu //

nādānusandhānkameva kāryaṃ
manyāmahe mānyatamaṃ layānāṃ // 12 //

The same opinion is endorsed in HP also—

Tr. *Śrī-ādinātha* has explained one crore and a quarter methods of *laya*. We consider *nādānusandhāna* as the most efficacious of all the *layas*. 12.

---

1. लययोगश्चित्तलयात्-N.2. लयः-n2,n3,n4,J . 3 . सार्धकोटिरुदीरितः-n2,n3,n4,J.
4 . शिर-T,n1. 5. तदेव-J,n1 . 6 . मत्सम्मतम्-P,T,t1, मत्स्येन्द्रमतं–J,n1.
7 . नादानुसन्धानमेकमेव-P,T,n1,t1, नादानुसन्धानमेव–N.

Note : *Saṅketa* is a technical term used here, which refers to the technique used for the absorption of the mind (*laya*). Although *Śrīnivāsa* refers to one and half crores of the techniques of *laya* (absorption of mind) and states that HP also quotes similarly, we find in HP (iv-66) the mention of one crore and a quarter types of absorption. 10-12.

लयो लय इति प्राहुः कीदृशं लयलक्षणम्[1] ||
अपुनर्भवसंस्थानं[2] लयो विषयविस्मृतिः || 13 ||
layo laya iti prāhuḥ kīdṛśaṃ layalakṣaṇam //
apunarbhavasaṃsthānaṃ layo viṣayavismṛtiḥ // 13 //

Tr. *Laya* has been emphasized. But what are the characteristics of *laya* ? *Laya* is not to come back to the world of senses. *Laya* is forgetting the objects of experience. 13.

अथ राजयोगः[3] —
न दृष्ट[4]लक्षाणि[5] न चित्तभंगो[6] न देशकालौ न च वायुरोधः ||
न धारणाध्यानपरिश्रमो वा समेधमाने सति राजयोगे || 14 ||

atha rājayogaḥ —
na dṛṣṭalakṣāṇi na cittabhaṅgo
na deśakālau na ca vāyurodhaḥ //
na dhāraṇādhyānapariśramo vā
samedhamāne sati rājayoge // 14 //

Tr. On attainment of the state of *rājayoga*, there remains no object for the eyes (senses), *citta* does not undergo further modification, one transcends time and space, there is no need to control the breath or undergo the hardship of practicing *dhāraṇā* and *dhyāna*. 14.

न जागरो नास्ति सुषुप्तिभावो न जीवितं[7] न[8] मरणं न[9] चित्तम्[10] ||
अहं ममत्वाद्यपहाय सर्वे[11] श्रीराजयोगस्थिरचेतनानाम् || 15 ||

---

1. कोटी वा लक्षणं-P, कोटीनां लयलक्षणं–J,n1,n2. 2. अपुनर्भावसंस्थाने-P, अपुनर्भा वसंस्थानं–T. 3. अथ भण्यते राजयोगः-P,T. 4. दृष्टि-P,J,T,n2,t1. 5. लक्ष्याणि-P,T,t1. 6. चित्तबन्धो-P,T,t1. 7. नाजीवितं -J. 8. नो –P,t1. 9. नामरणं न चित्तं-P,n1, 10. चित्रं–T. 11. सर्व –P,T,J,n1,n2,t1.

na jāgaro nāsti suṣuptibhāvo
na jīvitaṃ na maraṇaṃ na cittam //
ahaṃ mamatvādyapahāya sarve
śrīrājayogasthiracetanānām // 15 //

Tr. Those who attain the absolute state of consciousness through *rājayoga*, their *citta* does not experience awakening or sleep, living or dying states. They transcend the sense of 'I' and 'mine'. 15.

राजयोगं विना पृथ्वी राजयोगं विना निशा ॥
राजयोगं विना मुद्रा विचित्रापि न राजते[1] ॥ 16 ॥
rājayogaṃ vinā pṛthvī rājayogaṃ vinā niśā //
rājayogaṃ vinā mudrā vicitrāpi na rājate // 16 //

Tr. Without *rājayoga* as an objective, *āsanas* (*pṛthvī*) or *kumbhaka* (*niśā*) or even the amazing *mudrās* are useless. 16.

Note: This verse is the repetition of the verse from HP. The terms *pṛthvī, niśā* and *mudrā* have been used respectively for the *āsanas, prāṇāyāmas* and the *mudrās* or *karaṇas,* which form the curriculum of *haṭhayoga* and lead to the results of *rājayoga.* 16.

पीठानि कुम्भकाश्चित्रा दिव्यानि करणानि च ॥
सांगोऽपि[2] च हठाभ्यासो राजयोगफलार्थदः ॥ 17 ॥
pīṭhāni kumbhakāścitrā divyāni karaṇāni ca //
sāṅgo'pi ca haṭhābhyāso rājayogaphalārthadaḥ // 17 //

Tr. A consistent practice of the techniques of the *āsanas,* various *kumbhakas* and valuable *mudrās* which are the components of *haṭhayoga*, brings about success in *rājayoga*. 17.

अथ हठयोगः[3] —

महामुद्रादिदशकं कर्माण्यष्टौ च कुम्भकाः ॥
चतुरशीत्यासनानि[4] प्राहुश्चैतद्धठास्वयम् ॥ 18 ॥

---

1. जायते -J. 2. सर्वोपि –T,t1, संगोऽपि -P . 3. अथ श्री हठयोगः-P,T,t1.
4. चतुराशीत्यासनानि-P,t1.

atha haṭhayogaḥ —
mahāmudrādidaśakaṃ karmāṇyaṣṭau ca kumbhakāḥ //
caturaśītyāsanāni prāhuścaitaddhaṭhāhvayam // 18 //

Tr. The *haṭha* course of practices as propagated, comprises the ten *mudrās* like *mahāmudrā*, the eight *kriyās*, eight *kumbhakas* and eightyfour *āsanas*. 18.

हठं[1] विना राजयोगो राजयोगं विना हठः ||
व्याप्तिः स्यादविनाभूता श्रीराज[2]हठयोगयोः || 19 ||

haṭhaṃ vinā rājayogo rājayogaṃ vinā haṭhaḥ //
vyāptiḥ syādavinābhūtā śrīrājahaṭhayogayoḥ // 19 //

Tr. Without *haṭha*, *rājayoga* cannot be accomplished; so also without *rājayoga* as an objective, *haṭhayoga* cannot be perfected. Therefore, *rājayoga* and *haṭhayoga* are inter-dependent. 19.

Note: This verse describes mutual relationship and interdependance of *haṭhayoga* and *rājayoga*. 19.

मतान्तरे तु –
मकारेण मनः प्रोक्तं त्रकारः प्राण उच्यते ||
मनःप्राणसमायोगाद् योगो वै मन्त्रसञ्ज्ञकः || 20 ||

matāntare tu —
makāreṇa manaḥ proktaṃ trakāraḥ prāṇa ucyate //
manaḥprāṇasamāyogād yogo vai mantrasañjñakaḥ // 20 //

Another opinion —

Tr. '*Ma*' denotes mind, '*tra*' stands for '*prāṇa*'. *Mantrayoga* is the synthesis of '*manas*' and '*prāṇa*'. 20.

अपान[3]वृत्तिमाकृष्य प्राणो[4] गच्छति मध्यमे[5] ||
राजते गगनाम्भोजे राजयोगस्तु तेन वै || 21 ||

apānavṛttimākṛṣya prāṇo gacchati madhyame //
rājate gaganāmbhoje rājayogastu tena vai // 21 //

---

1. **हठ** –N. 2 . **श्रीराजं** – N. 3. **अपाण**-N. 4 . **प्राणं** – N,n1. 5 . **मध्यगं** – N,n1, **मध्यमं** -J.

Tr. By controlling the activity of *apāna, prāṇa* enters into the middle (*suṣumnā*). When it (*prāṇa*) is established into the space (*bramarandhra*), one attains *rājayoga*. 21.

हकारेणोच्यते सूर्यष्ठकारश्चन्द्रसञ्ज्ञकः[1] ॥
चन्द्रसूर्ये समीभूते हठश्च परमार्थदः[2] ॥ 22 ॥

hakāreṇocyate sūryaṣṭhakāraścandrasañjñakaḥ //
candrasūrye samībhūte haṭhaśca paramārthadaḥ // 22 //

Tr. '*Ha*' stands for *sūrya* (sun), while '*ṭha*' stands for *candra* (moon). When through *haṭha* (practices) *candra* and *sūrya* are unified, it yieds to liberation. 22.

युवा भवति वृद्धोऽपि[3] व्याधितो दुर्बलोऽपि वा ॥
अभ्यासात्सिद्धिमाप्नोति सर्वयोगेष्वतन्द्रितः ॥ 23 ॥

yuvā bhavati vṛddho'pi vyādhito durbalo'pi vā //
abhyāsāt siddhimāpnoti sarvayogeṣvatandritaḥ // 23 //

Tr. Through a diligent practice, one attains success in all the *yogas,* irrespective of one's being young, old, diseased or decrepit. 23.

अभ्यासकाले प्रथमे शस्तं क्षीरादिभोजनम् ॥
ततोऽभ्यासे दृढीभूते न तावन्नियमग्रहः[4] ॥ 24 ॥

abhyāsakāle prathame śastaṃ kṣīrādibhojanam //
tato'bhyāse dṛḍhībhūte na tāvanniyamagrahaḥ // 24 //

Tr. In the initial stage of practice, it is right to consume food prepared of milk and the like. As one gradually progresses, sticking to such food may not be necessary. 24.

अभ्यासकाले प्रथमे निषिञ्चन्ति कफादयः ॥
अकार्य[5]कर्मभावेन भविष्यन्त्यखिलामयाः ॥ 25 ॥

1.----चन्द्रसूचकः-P,T,t1. 2.--हठयोगोऽभिधीयते–P,T,t1. 3.वृद्धोवा-P,T,t1. 4.तावान्नियमग्रहः-P. 5.अर्कार्य -N.

abhyāsakāle prathame niṣiñcanti kaphādayaḥ //
akāryakarmabhāvena bhaviṣyantyakhilāmayāḥ // 25 //

Tr. In the first phase of practice, a practitioner should overcome phlegmatic disorders. If purificatory practices (*karmas*) are ignored, a host of diseases would result. 25.

अत्र वयं गुरुसम्प्रदायानुसारेण चक्र्याद्य[1]ष्ट-कर्माणि ब्रूमः—

चक्रि[2]नौलिर्धौतिनेतिबस्तिश्च[3] गजकरिणी[4] ॥
त्राटकं[5] मस्तकभ्रान्तिः[6] कर्माण्यष्टौ प्रचक्षते ॥ 26 ॥[7]

atra vayaṃ gurusampradāyānusāreṇa cakryādyaṣṭakarmāṇi brūmaḥ —

cakrinaulirdhautinetibastiśca gajakariṇī //
trāṭakaṃ mastakabhrāntiḥ karmāṇyaṣṭau pracakṣate // 26 //

Now we will narrate the eight karmas, (purificatory processes) like *cakri* etc., following the tradition of our *guru*—

Tr. The eight *karmas* are – *cakri, nauli, dhauti, neti, basti, gajakariṇī, trāṭaka* and *mastakabhrānti*. 26.

Note: In this verse *Śrīnivāsa* has mentioned eightfold cleansing processes according to his own tradition, in which *cakri-karma* is given great importance. 26.

हठप्रदीपिकायाम्[8] —

बस्तिर्धौति[9]स्तथा नेतिस्त्राटकं[10] नौलिकं[11] तथा ॥
कपालभ्रान्तिरेतानि[12] षट्कर्माणि प्रचक्षते ॥ 27 ॥

haṭhapradīpikāyām —

bastirdhautistathā netistrāṭakaṃ naulikaṃ tathā //
kapālabhrāntiretāni ṣaṭkarmāṇi pracakṣate // 27 //

According to *Haṭhapradīpikā*—

Tr. The *ṣaṭ-karmas* are – *basti, dhauti, neti, trāṭaka, naulika* and *kapāla-bhrānti*. 27.

Note : HP describes sixfold purificatory processes in

---

1. नौल्यादय-P,T,t1. 2. चक्रिर्-T,t1. गजकारिणी-N,T, गजधारिणी–J, 3. चक्रिनौलिधौतिर्ने तिर्वस्तिर्ग-जकरिणी–P. 4. नीतिबस्ति -T. 5. त्रोटनं-P, त्रौटनं -T. 6. मस्तकभातिः-P,n1, मस्तकं भ्रान्तिः-J. 7. अनुपलब्धश्लोकः-n1. 8. स्वात्मारामनते तु' - अधिकपाठः-P,T,t1. 9. धौतिर्वस्ति–P,J,T,t1. 10. स्त्रटकं–P, नीतिः त्रोटकं-T. 11. नौलिका -P,T,t1. 12. कपालभ्रान्तिश्चैतानि –P,T,t1.

which*cakri-karma* is not mentioned, to which *Śrīnivāsa* has taken a great objection and criticised about his ignorance. Although, HP talks about sixfold purificatory processes, it also describes *gajakaraṇī* in addition to the six processes. *Śrīnivāsa* quotes HP and mentions *kapālabhrānti* instead of *kapālabhāti*, which we get in most of the copies of HP. *Śrīnivāsa* uses the term *mastakabhrānti* as a synonym for widely used term *kapālabhāti*. In the HP text with 10 chapters (iii. 23), we also get another term as *kapālabhastrī*. 27.

इदं मतं चिन्तनीयं चक्र्यभावे[1] कथं भवेत् ? उद्देश्यस्य विरोधित्वादसंगतमिदं मतम् | हठप्रदीपिकोक्तदूषण[2]निराकरणप्रयासस्तु उत्तुंगशृंग-वपुर्भग'- प्रसंगमनुकरोति[3] | अलं नखच्छेद्ये[4] परशु[5]प्रहारेणेत्युपरम्यते |

idaṃ mataṃ cintanīyaṃ cakryabhāve kathaṃ bhavet ? uddeśyasya virodhitvādasaṅgatamidaṃ matam / haṭhapradīpikoktadūṣaṇa nirākaraṇaprayāsastu ' uttuṅgaśṛṅga-vapurbhaṅga ' prasaṅgamanukaroti / alaṃ nakhacchedye paraśu-prahāreṇetyuparamyate //

Tr. How can this opinion be accepted without *cakrī* ? This is inappropriate as it contradicts the very purpose. To counteract the faulty opinion expressed in HP is like 'breaking ones own limbs in an attempt to climb a lofty mountain'. One need not use an axe to trim the nails.

कर्माष्टकमिदं गोप्यं घटशोधनकारकम् ||
कस्यचिन्नैव वक्तव्यं कुलस्त्रीसुरतं यथा || 28 ||

karmāṣṭakamidaṃ gopyaṃ ghaṭaśodhanakārakam //
kasyacinnaiva vaktavyaṃ kulastrīsuratam yathā // 28 //

Tr. The eight *karmas* are to be kept secret, as they are effective in cleansing the body (*ghaṭa*). These should not be disclosed to anybody, like a noble woman who would not disclose her sexual pleasures to anybody. 28.

1.चक्र्यभावं -P. 2. दूषणानि– P,T. 3 .उत्तुंगर्शृग प्रसंगमनुकरोति -N,T. 4. नखछेदे – J,N,n1. 5. पर्शु–N,n1.

अथ चक्रिकर्म[1] —
पायुनाले प्रसार्यार्द्धमंगुलीं [2] भ्रामयेदभीः ॥
यावद् गुद[3]विकासः स्याच्चक्रिकर्म निगद्यते ॥ 29 ॥

***atha cakrikarma*—**
pāyunāle prasāryārddhamaṅgulīṃ bhrāmayedabhīḥ //
yāvad gudavikāsaḥ syāccakrikarma nigadyate // 29 //

Tr. One should insert the half-length of the finger in the anus by opening it and move the finger round until the anal sphincters are fully relaxed. This is *cakri-karma*. 29.

Note: SKS(15) describes three kinds of *cakri*, namely, *ūrdhva-cakri*, *madhya-cakri* and *adhaścakri*. The *cakri-karma* described here represents *adhaścakri* of SKS(37-38).

This process of *cakri-karma* is described as *mūlaśodhana* in GhS (I.41-42). 29.

मूलव्याधिः गुल्मरोगो[4] नश्यत्यत्र महोदरः ॥
मलशुद्ध्युद्दीपनं[5] च जायते चक्रिकर्मणा ॥ 30 ॥

mūlavyādhiḥ gulmarogo naśyatyatra mahodaraḥ //
malaśuddhyuddīpanaṃ ca jāyate cakrikarmaṇā // 30 //

Tr. Practice of *cakri-karma* removes the diseases like piles, (enlargement of) spleen and abdominal disorders, cleanses the morbidities and stimulates gastric fire. 30.

सर्वेषां कर्मणां[6] चक्रिसाधनं[7] प्रोच्यते मया ॥
स्वात्मारामप्रभूणां तु चक्रिकर्म न सम्मतम् ॥ 31 ॥

sarveṣāṃ karmaṇāṃ cakrisādhanaṃ procyate mayā //
svātmārāmaprabhūṇāṃ tu cakrikarma na sammatam // 31 //

Tr. Among all the *karmas*, I emphasise practice of *cakri-karma*. Learned *Svātmārāma* does not approve of *cakri-karma*.31.

---

1. अनुपलब्धपाठः–N,J,n1,n2. 2. मंगुलिं-T. 3. यावद् दृढ-N,J,T,n1. 4. गुल्मरोगौ–T. 5. मलशुद्धिर्दीपनं-P,N,t1. 6. कर्मचक्राणां-N,J,T,n1, कर्मचक्रिसाधनं–n2. 7. कर्मचक्राणां साधनं–N.

साधकैस्तत्[1] प्रकर्तव्यं[2] सर्वकर्माभिसिद्धये[3] ॥
तस्मान्मदुक्तरीत्यैव ज्ञातव्यं योगिपुंगवैः ॥ 32 ॥

sādhakaistat prakartavyaṃ sarvakarmābhisiddhaye //
tasmānmaduktarītyaiva jñātavyaṃ yogipuṅgavaiḥ // 32 //

Tr. To attain success in all the *karmas*, the practioners should follow the technique as laid down by me, which may also be noted by the eminent *yogīs*. 32.

अथ नौलिः—
सा च नौलिर्द्विधा प्रोक्ता भारी चैकान्तराभिधा[4] ॥
भारी स्याद् बाह्यरूपेण जायन्तेऽन्तस्तु सा तथा[5] ॥ 33 ॥

atha nauliḥ —
sā ca naulirdvidhā proktā bhārī caikāntarābhidhā //
bhārī syād bāhyarūpeṇa jāyante'ntastu sā tathā // 33 //

Tr. *Bhārī* and *antarā* are the two varieties of *nauli*. *Bhārī* is external, while the *antarā* is internal. 33.

[6]अमन्दावर्तवेगेन तुन्दं[7] सव्यापसव्यतः ॥
नतांसो भ्रामयेदेषा[8] नौलिः गौडैः[9] प्रशस्यते[10] ॥ 34 ॥

amandāvartavegena tundaṃ savyāpasavyataḥ //
natāṃso bhrāmayedeṣā nauliḥ gauḍaiḥ praśasyate // 34 //

Tr. One rapidly rotates the abdomen to right and left (clockwise) and left to right (anti-clockwise) while bending down the shoulders. According to the *gauḍa*, this great practice is *nauli*. 34

तुन्दाग्निसन्दीपनपाचनादि[11]सन्दीपिकाऽऽनन्दकरी सदैव[12] ॥
अशेषदोषामयशोषिणी[13] च हठक्रियामौलिरियं च[14] नौलिः ॥ 35 ॥
tundāgnisandīpanapācanādi-sandīpikā'nandakarī sadaiva /
aśeṣadoṣāmayaśoṣiṇī ca haṭhakriyāmauliriyaṃ ca nauliḥ 35

---

1 . साधकैस्तत्र-P,T,t1. 2 . कर्तव्यं-P,T,t1. 3 . सर्वकर्मापि सिद्धये-P,T,t1. 4 . चैकान्तिकान्तरा-P. 5.जायते तथा–J, जायते गुन्द्र सा तथा–N,n1. 6. अथ बाह्याख्या नौलिः -P, अथ भार्याख्या नौलिः-T,n2. 7 . गुदं–J,N. 8. भ्रामयत्येषा–P, भ्रामयेदेषां–T,t1. 9 . गौड-N. 10. भ्रामयेच्चैष नौलिगौडः प्रशस्यत–J. . 11 . पाचनानि-N,J. 12. तदैव–T. 13 ..... शोषणी-P,T,t1. 14 . हि–J.

Tr. This *nauli* is the crown of all the *haṭha-kriyās,* which stimulates gastric fire, improves digestion, brings about a deep sense of well-being and completely removes all the disorders caused by vitiation of the three humours. 35.

अथ अन्तरा —
इडया[1]वर्तवेगेन[2] तथा पिंगलया पुनः ॥
उभाभ्यां भ्रामयेच्चैव[3] ह्यन्तरा कीर्तिता मया ॥ 36 ॥

atha antarā —
iḍayāvartavegena tathā piṅgalayā punaḥ //
ubhābhyāṃ bhrāmayeccaiva hyantarā kīrtitā mayā / 36 /

Tr. Quick rotation (of the abdomen) like a whirlpool on both sides, with the *idā* (left), followed by *piṅgalā* (right) is called *antarā* by me. 36.

Note : GhS (i.51) uses the term *laulikī* for *nauli.* HP describes only one type of *nauli.* Here two types of *nauli* have been described, namely, *bhārī* and *antarā.* We do not come across these terms elsewhere. SKS (110-114) describes different varieties of *nauli* such as *bāhya-nauli, nāla-nauli, āntra-nauli.* Although *śrīnivāsa* describes two types of *nauli* such as *bhārī* and *antarā,* the difference between the two is not clear. The terms *āntranauli* and *antarānauli* seem to have similarity. But the technique of *āntranauli* has been clearly described by SKS (114). The description of *antarānauli* by *Śrīnivāsa* does not show any difference in the technique of *bhārīnauli* and *antarānauli*, except the use of different terms like *savyāpasavyataḥ* and *iḍayā piṅgalayā.* Both these terms indicate the same process of rotating the nauli clockwise and anticlockwise. *Nauli* was one of the first *haṭhayogic* practices subjected to scientific investigation by Swāmī Kuvalayānanda in 1920s. It is now known that high sub-atmospheric pressure (partial vacuum) is created in all the cavities of the abdomen during *nauli.* The discovery of partial vacuum in the colon during *nauli* was named '*Mādhavadāsa* vacuum' by Swāmī Kuvalayānanda. For scientific studies on *nauli,* refer to YM vol. 1. 33-36.

---

1. ईड्या–T, इडाया –t1. 2. हठायावर्त्तवेगेन–T. 3. भ्रामयेश्चैषा–P, भ्रामणेश्चैषा–T.

अथ धौतिः —
विंशद्धस्तप्रमाणेन धौतवस्त्रं[1] सुदीर्घितम् ॥
चतुरंगुलविस्तारं सिक्तं चैव शनैः[2] ग्रसेत् ॥ 37 ॥
ततः प्रत्याहरेच्चैतदभ्यासाद्[3]द्धौतिरुच्यते ॥
दिने दिने ततः कुर्याज्जठराग्निः प्रवर्द्धते[4] ॥ 38 ॥
atha dhautiḥ —
viṃśaddhastapramāṇena dhautavastraṃ sudīrghitam //
caturaṅgulavistāraṃ siktaṃ caiva śanaiḥ graset // 37 //
tataḥ pratyāhareccaitadabhyāsāddhautirucyate //
dine dine tataḥ kuryājjaṭharāgniḥ pravarddhate //38 //

Tr. One should slowly swallow a clean wet cloth measuring twenty cubits in length and four digits in width, and thereafter pull the same out. This is called *dhauti*, which has to be mastered over day by day. This enhances gastric fire. 37-38.

कासश्वासप्लीहकुष्ठं[5] कफरोगाश्च[6] विंशतिः ॥
धौतिकर्मप्रभावेन धावन्त्येव[7] न संशयः ॥ 39 ॥
kāsaśvāsaplīhakuṣṭhaṃ kapharogāśca viṃśatiḥ //
dhautikarmaprabhāvena dhāvantyeva na saṃśayaḥ // 39 //

Tr. Practice of *dhauti* undoubtedly removes the diseases like cough, asthma, spleen (disorders), skin diseases and all the twenty varieties of phlegmatic disorders. 39.

Note : The length of the cloth for *dhauti* seems to vary in different traditions. HP(ii.24) describes the length of the cloth to be 15 cubits, while HSC suggests the measure to be anywhere between 15 to 20 cubits. GhS(I.39), however, suggests it to be between 19 to 25 cubits. This form of *dhauti* is generally considered as *vastradhauti*. GhS (i.35) considers *vastra-dhauti* under the category of *hṛd-dhauti.*

---

1. धौतेर्वस्त्र-P,T,t1. 2. शनैः शनैः-T. 3. प्रत्याहरेच्चौदुत्खातं-P,T,n2.. 4. जठराग्निप्रवर्धनम्-P,T,n1,n2,t1. 5. कुष्ठ–n1,n2,n3,n4,P,T. 6 ....कफरोगोष्म - P,T,t1. 7. धावत्येव–J.

GhS(i.13-14) also elaborately describes *dhauti* into 13 types, which we do not find elsewhere.

Vastra-dhauti has been found greatly efficacious in the treatment of respiratory and metabolic disorders like asthma, obesity etc. For scientific experiments on *dhauti,* refer to YM vol. 2, pp. 168-195 and vol. 11, pp. 9-14. 37-39.

अथ नेतिकर्म[1] —

आखुपुच्छाकारनिभं सूत्रं सुस्निग्धनिर्मितम् ||
षड्वितस्तिमितं[2] सूत्रं नेति[3]सूत्रस्य लक्षणम् || 40 ||

atha netikarma —

ākhupucchākāranibhaṃ sūtraṃ susnigdhanirmitam //
ṣaḍvitastimitaṃ sūtraṃ netisūtrasya lakṣaṇam // 40 //

Tr. A sheaf of smooth cotton thread resembling the tail of a mouse, which is six *vitasti* (1 *vitasti* = 12 digits) in length, is the characteristic of the thread used for *neti.* 40.

नासानाले प्रविश्यैनं मुखान्निर्गमयेत् क्रमात् ||
सूत्रस्यान्तं[4] प्रबद्ध्वा तु[5] भ्रामयेन्नासनालयोः ||
मथनं[6] च ततः कुर्यान्नेतिः[7] सिद्धैर्निगद्यते || 41 ||

nāsānāle praviśyainaṃ mukhānnirgamayet kramāt //
sūtrasyāntaṃ prabaddhvā tu bhrāmayennāsanālayoḥ //
mathanaṃ ca tataḥ kuryānnetiḥ siddhairnigadyate // 41 /

Tr. Insert it in one of the nostrils and pull it out through the mouth. By holding the ends of the thread and tying their ends, it should be rotated in the nasal passage and given friction. According to *siddhas,* this is *neti.* 41.

कपालशोधिनी[8] कार्या[9] दिव्यदृष्टिप्रदायिनी ||
जत्रूर्ध्वजातरोगघ्नी[10] जायते नेतिरुत्तमा[11] || 42 ||[12]

---

1. अथ नेति–n1, अथ नीतिकर्म—T,n2. 2. षड्वित्तनिर्मितं -N,J,n1, षड्विधस्तिमितं - T. 3. नीति-N,J,T,n1,n2,t1. 4. सूत्रा . . – J. 5. प्रवर्द्धन्तु-N,n1,J, प्रबध्वाशु -T. 6. मन्थनं–n1,t1. 7. कुर्या-न्नीति-N,n1,J,T,t1. 8. कपालशोधनी-P,T. 9. चैव–P, कण्ठ्या-T. 10. जत्रूर्ध्वजातरोगघ्ना–P,T,t1. 11. नीतिरुत्तमा-N,J,T,t1. 12. अनन्तरं 'नेतिस्वरूपं कथितं श्रीनिवासेन योगिना' अधिकपाठः-P, अनन्तरं 'नीतिस्वरूपं कथितं श्रीनिवासेन योगिना' अधिकपाठः-T,t1.

kapālaśodhinī kāryā divyadṛṣṭipradāyinī //
jatrūrdhvajātarogaghnī jāyate netiruttamā // 42 //

Tr. This excellent practice cleanses the frontal sinuses, offers keen eyesight and removes the diseases above the neck. 42.

Note: The word *neti* refers to a smooth sheaf of cotton having different lengths used for purification of the nasal cavity. HP(ii-30) describes the length of it measuring approximately 23 cms. This process is popularly known as *sūtra-neti*. SKS (68) mentions two types of *neti* distinguished by the thread rolled and not rolled. The technique described by *Śrīnivāsa* is different from the generally known technique. It resembles *netri-karaṇa* described in SKS (44-45).

The purpose of *neti* is not only to cleanse the nasal passage, but also to render the nasal mucus membrane resistant to the environmental changes. 40-42.

अथ बस्तिः[1] —
बस्तिस्तु द्विविधो[2] प्रोक्तः[3] जलवायुप्रभेदतः ॥
चक्रिं कृत्वा यथाशक्त्या बस्तिञ्चैव तु कारयेत् ॥ 43 ॥
atha bastiḥ —
bastistu dvividho proktaḥ jalavāyuprabhedataḥ //
cakriṃ kṛtvā yathāśaktyā bastiñcaiva tu kārayet // 43 //

Tr. *Basti* is of two types: *vāyu-basti* and *jala-basti*. After practising *cakri*, one must undertake the practice of *basti*. 43.

Note: It is to be noted that *Śrīnivāsa* recommends the practice of *cakrikarma* before the practice of *basti*. 43.

वायुमाकुञ्च्य जठरे गुदनाले विसर्जयेत् ॥
वायुबस्तिरियं प्रोक्ता[4] जलबस्तिमथ[5] ब्रुवे[6] ॥ 44 ॥

vāyumākuñcya jaṭhare gudanāle visarjayet //
vāyubastiriyaṃ proktā jalabastimatha bruve // 44 //

---

1. अथ बस्तिकर्म-J,n1. 2. द्विविधा –P,J,N,n1,T,t1. 3. प्रोक्ता–J,N,n1,P,T,t1. 4. प्रोक्तं –T,t1. 5. मथो–n1,t1. 6 जलबस्तिमथोच्यते-T.

अथ हठप्रदीपिकाकारमते तु[1] —
नाभिदघ्नजले पायुं[2] न्यस्त[3]नालोत्कटासनः ॥
आधाराकुञ्चनं[4] कुर्यात् कापालं बस्तिकर्म तत् ॥ 50 ॥

atha haṭhapradīpikākāramate tu —
nābhidaghnajale pāyuṃ nyastanālotkaṭāsanaḥ //
ādhārākuñcanaṃ kuryāt kāpālaṃ bastikarma tat // 50 //

According to the author of HP —

Tr. One adopts *utkaṭāsana* in navel-deep water. After inserting a tube in the anus, one manipulates the anus to raise the water upwards. This is *kāpāla-basti-karma.* 50.

अस्माकं तु पायुन्यस्तनालेन[5] जलाकुञ्चनमेकदेशयोगीन्द्रमार्गबस्तिकर्म प्रकारापेक्षया पायुनाले[6] न्यस्ताङ्गुल्या[7] आकुञ्च्य जलबस्तिमार्गः[8] चर्पट्यादि[9]सर्व योगीन्द्रसाधारणो अयमेव प्रकारः समीचीन इव प्रतिभाति ॥

asmākaṃ tu pāyunyastanālena jalākuñcanamekadeśa-yogīndra-mārga-bastikarma-prakārāpekṣayā pāyunāle nyastāṅgulyā ākuñcya jalabastimārgaḥ carpaṭyādisarvayogīndrasādhāraṇo ayameva prakāraḥ samīcīna iva pratibhāti //

Tr. We hold that instead of insertion of a tube in the anal canal and drawing the water through the tube in the *basti-karma* as practised by some adepts of *yoga,* one should practise *jala-basti* by inserting the finger in the anus, which was widely accepted by all eminent *yogīs* like *Carpaṭi* etc. This (latter) version seems to be the proper one.

अथ गजकरणी[10] —
उदरगतपदार्थमुद्वमन्ती[11] पवनमपानमुदीर्य कण्ठनाले ॥
क्रमपरिचयतस्तु[12] वायुमार्गे गजकरणीति[13] निगद्यते हठज्ञैः ॥ 51 ॥

---

1. हठप्रदीपिकामते तु–J,n2. 2. पायुः-P, पायु -T. 3. न्यस्ता–J. 4. आधारकुंचनं -P,T. 5. पायुन्यस्तनाले -P,T,t1. 6. पायुनाल–P,T,t1. 7. न्यस्तांगुलया –P. 8. मार्ग –N,n1,J. 9. यथेछादि –N,J. 10. गजकरिणी -N. 11 ....मुद्वहंत्या –N,n1,J. 12. क्रमपरिचरितस्तु –N. 13. गजकरिणी –N, गजकरणी- P.

atha gajakaraṇī —
udaragatapadārthamudvamantī
pavanamapānamudīrya kaṇṭhanāle //
kramaparicayatastu vāyumārge
gajakaraṇīti nigadyate haṭhajñaiḥ // 51 //

Tr. One vomits the contents of the stomach by stimulating and raising the *apāna-vāyu* upto the throat, through a gradual practice of gaining control over the passage of the air. The experts of *haṭha* call this *gajakaraṇī.* 51.

Note: This verse has the similarity of the verse in HP (ii.26). 51.

अथवा —
पीत्वाऽऽकण्ठं सतिलगुडजलं[1] नालिकेरोदकं वा
[2]वायुमार्गे पवनजलयुतं[3] कुम्भयेद्वाथ शक्त्या ॥
निःशेषं शोधयित्वा परिभवपवनो[4] बस्तिवायुप्रकाशात्[5]
कुम्भाम्भः कण्ठनाले गुरुगजकरणी[6] प्रोच्यतेऽयं हठज्ञैः ॥ 52 ॥

athavā —
pītvā'kaṇṭhaṃ satilaguḍajalaṃ nālikerodakaṃ vā
vāyumārge pavanajalayutaṃ kumbhayedvātha śaktyā/
niḥśeṣaṃ śodhayitvā paribhavapavano bastivāyuprakāśāt
kumbhāmbhaḥ kaṇṭhanāle gurugajakaraṇī -
procyate'yaṃ haṭhajñaiḥ // 52 //

Moreover—

Tr. One should drink water mixed up with jaggery and sesame or coconut water up to the throat and retain both water and air to the limit. With an objective to control '*pavana*', one should thoroughly cleanse the whole tract from stomach to the throat. This is called *guru-gajakaraṇī*, by the experts of *haṭha.* 52.

---

1. पीत्वाकंदंमतिजलल-N,n1, सतिगुडजलं –t1, पीत्वाकण्ठं सति –P,T. 2. पूर्व 'क्षीराम्भो' अधिकपाठः-P,T,t1. 3. युतः -T,t1. 4. शोधयेद्वापरिभवनमनो–N,n1,J. 5. वस्तिवायुप्रकारात् -J,N,n1. 6. गजकरण इति–N,n1, J.

Note: The technique of *gajakaraṇī* described here is called *guru-gajakaraṇī,* which requires drinking of coconut water or the water mixed with jaggery and sesame. This technique is not found described elsewhere. 52.

यथैव गजयूथानां[1] राजते राजकुञ्जरः ॥
तथैव हठतन्त्राणां मुख्या हि गजकरिणी[2] ॥ 53 ॥

yathaiva gajayūthānāṃ rājate rājakuñjaraḥ //
tathaiva haṭhatantrāṇāṃ mukhyā hi gajakariṇī // 53 //

Tr. As the leader of the elephants shines among the herd of the elephants, similarly, *gajakariṇī* is the foremost among the *haṭha* practices. 53.

अथ त्राटकम्[3] —
निरीक्ष्य निश्चलदृशा सूक्ष्मलक्ष्यं समाहितः[4] ॥
अश्रुसम्पातपर्यन्तमाचार्यैस्त्राटकं[5] स्मृतम् ॥ 54 ॥

atha trāṭakaṃ —
nirīkṣya niścaladṛśā sūkṣmalakṣyaṃ samāhitaḥ //
aśrusampātaparyantamācāryaistrāṭakaṃ smṛtam // 54 //

Tr. One should constantly gaze at a very minute object, remaining one-pointed, until tears roll down. According to the adepts, this is *trāṭaka.* 54.

स्फोटनं नेत्ररोगाणां तन्द्रादीनां[6] कपाटकम्[7] ॥
प्रयत्नात्त्राटकं [8] गोप्यं यथा रत्नसुपेटकम्[9] ॥ 55 ॥

sphoṭanaṃ netrarogāṇāṃ tandrādīnāṃ kapāṭakam //
prayatnāt-trāṭakaṃ gopyaṃ yathā ratnasupeṭakam // 55 //

Tr. This technique removes eye diseases drowsiness and the like. Therefore, it should be carefully guarded like a casket of jewels. 55.

---

1. गजयूधानां-T,t1. 2. गजकारिणी-n1,T,t1. 3. त्रोटकं-P,t1; त्रोटनं-T. 4. समीहितः-T. 5. ...त्रोटकं-P,T. 6. तन्द्राणां तु-n1,n2,n3,n4,J. 7. कवाटकम्-P,T,t1. 8. त्रोटनं-t1. 9. 'प्रयत्ला त्राटक पेटकं'–N,J,n1,n2, रत्नं सुपेटकं –P,T,t1.

Note: In some copies of Mss, instead of *trāṭaka*, the term *troṭaka* and *troṭana* are used. The technique of *trāṭaka* described in SKS (40-41) requires the *bījamantra vaṃ* and *glauṃ* to be accompanied during this process for the manifestation of the inner light. 55.

अथ कपालभस्त्रिका[1] –
भस्त्रिवल्लोहकाराणां रेचपूरससम्भ्रमौ ॥
कपालभस्त्री[2] विख्याता सर्वरोगविशोषणी ॥ 56 ॥

***atha kapālabhastrikā* –**
bhastrivallohakārāṇāṃ recapūrasusambhramau //
kapālabhastrī vikhyātā sarvarogaviśoṣaṇī // 56 //

Tr. One should rapidly inhale and exhale like the bellows of an ironsmith. This is the famous *kapāla-bhastrī*, which removes all the diseases. 56.

अथवा –
कपालं भ्रामयेत्सव्यमपसव्यं[3] तु वेगतः ॥
रेचपूरकयोगेन[4] कपालभस्त्रिरुच्यते[5] ॥ 57 ॥
***athavā* –**
kapālaṃ bhrāmayetsavyamapasavyaṃ tu vegataḥ //
recapūrakayogena kapālabhastrirucyate // 57 //
Or,

Tr. One moves the head quickly on right and left by inhalation and exhalation. This is *kapālabhastri*. 57.

Note: This process of *kapālabhastrī* or *kapālabhastrikā* has been termed as *kapālabhrānti* earlier in i. 27. The term *kapālabhrānti* seems appropriate with the technique given in i.57, where forceful and rapid exhalations and inhalations are accompanied with the movement of the head on left and right. SKS (50-54) calls this process as *bhastrā* and describes it of three kinds,namely, *shtirabhastrā, bhrāntibhastrā* and *antarbhastrā.* The technique

---

1. कपालभातिः-P; कपालभ्रान्त्रिः-T,t1. 2. कपालभ्रान्तिः-P,T,t1. 3. भ्रामयेत्सर्वमपसव्यं-T. 4. रेचपूर्व-कमुक्तेन-T,t1,P, रेचपूरकयुक्तेन–J. 5. कपालभ्रान्तिरुच्यते-T,t1,P.

of *bhrāntibhastrā* resembles the technique given here by *Śrīnivāsa*.

GhS(i.54) describes this process under *kapālabhāti* and gives three varieties of it, namely, *vātakrama, vyutkrama* and *śītkrama*. The *vātakrama kapālabhāti* requires the use of alternate nostrils. This variety is used in *bhastrikā prāṇāyāma*. The *vyutkrama kapālabhāti* and *śītkrama kapālabhāti* are done with water. In *vyutkrama kapālabhāti*, the water is drawn through the nose and expelled through the mouth, while in *śītkrama kapālabhāti*, the water is taken through the mouth and expelled through the nose.

Sundaradeva, the author of HSC, calls *vyutkrama kapālabhāti* as *śaṅkhaprakṣālana*, in which the water is drawn through one nostril and expelled through the other nostril. Popularly, this is known as *jalaneti*. In SKS(55), it is called *nāsādanti*. 57.

कफदोषं निहन्त्येव[1] पित्तदोषं जलोद्भवम् ॥
कपालशोधनञ्चापि[2] ब्रह्मचक्रं विशुद्ध्यति[3] ॥ 58 ॥

इत्यष्टकर्माणि[4] ॥

kaphadoṣaṃ nihantyeva pittadoṣaṃ jalodbhavam //
kapālaśodhanañcāpi brahmacakraṃ viśudhyati // 58 //

ityaṣṭakarmāṇi.

Tr. This practice alleviates the phlegmatic and bilious disorders and diseases caused due to water like (pleurisy etc.). Moreover, it cleanses the forehead and *brahmacakra*. 58.

Thus end the eight *karmas*.

वपुः[5]कृशत्वं वदने प्रसन्नता
नाद[6]स्फुटत्वं नयने च निर्मले[7] ॥
अरोगता बिन्दुजयोऽग्निदीपनं
नाडीषु शुद्धि[8]र्हठसिद्धिलक्षणम् ॥ 59 ॥

---

1. निहत्येव–J. 2. कपालशोधनंवापि-N,n1,T,t1,J. 3. विशु–N, विशुध्यते–J,n1, विशोध्यति–P,T. 4. इत्यष्टकर्मनिरूपणम्-P,T, इत्यष्टकर्म -J,n2. 5. वपु –N. 6. नादे – N,n1,J. 7. निर्मलं –N,n1. 8. सिद्धि -P,T,t1.

vapuḥkṛśatvaṃ vadane prasannatā
nādasphuṭatvaṃ nayane ca nirmale //
arogatā bindujayo'gnidīpanaṃ
nāḍīṣu śuddhirhaṭhasiddhilakṣaṇam // 59 //

Tr. The signs of success in *haṭhayoga* are:— slimness of the body, cheerful face, hearing of the mystical sound, shining eyes, a sense of wellness, control over the *bindu*, increase in gastric fire and purification of the *nāḍīs.* 59.

Note: This verse is similar to the verse of HP (ii.78). 59.

कर्माष्टभिर्गतस्थौल्यं[1] कफमेदोमलादिकम्[2] ॥
प्राणायामं ततः कुर्यादनायासेन सिद्ध्यति ॥ 60 ॥
karmāṣṭabhirgatasthaulyaṃ kaphamedomalādikam //
prāṇāyāmaṃ tataḥ kuryādanāyāsena siddhyati // 60 //

Tr. After removing the impurities, such as fat and phlegm, through the practice of the eight *karmas*, one should undertake the practice of *prāṇāyāma*, which is easily accomplished. 60.

षट्चक्रशोधनं सम्यक् प्राणायामस्य कारणम् ॥
नाशनं सर्वरोगाणां मोक्षमार्गस्य[3] साधनम् ॥ 61 ॥

ṣaṭcakraśodhanaṃ samyak prāṇāyāmasya kāraṇam //
nāśanaṃ sarvarogāṇāṃ mokṣamārgasya sādhanam // 61 //

Tr. (As a result of these eight *karmas*) the practice of *prāṇāyāma* becomes succeesful, all the six *cakras* are properly purified, all the diseases are removed, and liberation is achieved.61.

देहारोग्यं च लभते ह्यष्टकर्मप्रभावतः ॥
आधारशोधनं चक्र्या लिंगं वज्रोलिकर्मणा[4] ॥ 62 ॥

dehārogyaṃ ca labhate hyaṣṭakarmaprabhāvataḥ //
ādhāraśodhanaṃ cakryā liṅgaṃ vajrolikarmaṇā // 62 //

---

1. कर्माष्ट निर्गतं स्थौल्यं –N,n1. 2. कफमेदोमलाधिकः-P; कफमेदोमलादिकः-T,t1.
3. मोक्षकर्मस्य-T,t1. 4. वरयोलिकर्मणा-T.

Tr. As a result of *aṣṭa-karmas*, one gains physical wellness. *cakri-karma* purifies the *ādhāra,* while *vajrolī-karma* cleanses the generative organ. 62.

मणिपूरं नाभिगतं नौल्याख्येन तु कर्मणा ॥
हृदयं कण्ठचक्रं[1] च धौत्याख्येन तु कर्मणा ॥ 63 ॥

maṇipūraṃ nābhigataṃ naulyākhyena tu karmaṇā //
hṛdayaṃ kaṇṭhacakraṃ ca dhautyākhyena tu karmaṇā 63

Tr. *Nauli-karma* brings purification to *maṇipūra* located at the navel. *dhauti-karma* purifies the *hṛdaya cakra* and *kaṇṭha-cakra* at the throat. 63.

शोधनं कार्यमाज्ञायां नेतित्राटककर्मणा[2] ॥
सर्वांगशोधनं कार्यं बस्तिभस्त्रैककर्मणा[3] ॥ 64 ॥

śodhanaṃ kāryamājñāyāṃ netitrāṭakakarmaṇā //
sarvāṅgaśodhanaṃ kāryaṃ bastibhastraikakarmaṇā /64/

Tr. *Ājñā-cakra* is purified by *neti* and *trāṭaka-karmas.* Entire body is purified by *basti* and *bhastrā-karma* (*kapālabhāti*). 64.

स्यादाधारं स्वाधिष्ठानं मणिपूरमनाहतम् ॥
विशुद्धं कण्ठचक्रस्थमाज्ञाचक्रं भ्रुवोर्मुखे ॥[4]
चक्रभेदमिति ज्ञात्वा चक्रातीतं[5] निरञ्जनम् ॥ 65 ॥

syādādhāraṃ svādhiṣṭhānaṃ maṇipūramanāhatam //
viśuddhaṃ kaṇṭhacakrasthamājñācakraṃ bhruvormukhe/
cakrabhedamiti jñātvā cakrātītaṃ nirañjanam // 65 //

Tr. *Ādhāra, svādhiṣṭhāna, maṇipūra, anāhata, viśuddha* in the throat and *ājñā-cakra* at the center of the eyebrows—is the scheme of *cakras,* which one should know. *nirañjana*—the Absolute—is beyond (the ambit) of *cakras.* 65.

---

1. कण्ठचक्रस्थं-P,T,t1. 2. नेतित्रोटनकर्मणा-P, नीतिस्त्राटककर्मणा–J, नीतित्राटककर्मणा–N,n1, कार्य-माज्ञायामिति त्रोटनकर्मणा –t1. 3. वस्तिभस्त्रिककर्मणा -P,T,t1. 4. पंक्ति अनुपलब्धा –N, विशुद्धचक्राज्ञाचक्रे .... J,n1. 5. चकातीत -P,N.

Note: Note the purpose of *karmas* given here as purification of the six *cakras*. This is a special contribution of the *karmas* highlighted by the author. 61-65.

सुराष्ट्रे धार्मिके देशे सुभिक्षे निरुपद्रवे ॥
एकान्तमठिकामध्ये[1] स्थातव्यं हठयोगिना ॥ 66 ॥

surāṣṭre dhārmike deśe subhikṣe nirupadrave //
ekāntamaṭhikāmadhye sthātavyaṃ haṭhayoginā // 66 //

Tr. A practioner of *haṭhayoga* should reside in a peaceful righteous country, which is free from troubles and where alms are easily available. He should stay alone in a small cottage. 66.

अल्पद्वारमरन्ध्रगर्तपिठरं[2] नात्युच्चनीचायतम्
सम्यग्गोमयसान्द्रलिप्तविमलं निःशेषबाधोज्झितम् ॥
बाह्ये मण्डप[3] वेदिकूपरुचिरं[4] प्राकारसंवेष्टितम्[5]
प्रोक्तं योगमठस्य लक्षणमिदं सिद्धैर्हठाभ्यासिभिः ॥ 67 ॥

alpadvāramarandhragartapiṭharaṃ nātyuccanīcāyataṃ
samyaggomayasāndraliptavimalaṃ niḥśeṣabādhojjhitam //
bāhye maṇḍapavedikūparuciraṃ prākārasaṃveṣṭitam
proktaṃ yogamaṭhasya
lakṣaṇamidaṃ siddhairhaṭhābhyāsibhiḥ //67 //

Tr. According to the experts of *haṭhayoga*, an ideal cottage for *yoga* practice should have a small entrance, having no pits or holes, not too high or low, nicely smeared with a paste of cow dung, clean and free from all insects, having a canopied platform outside and a well (with pure water) and a fencing wall around. 67.

एवंविधे मठे स्थित्वा सर्वचिन्ताविवर्जितः ॥
गुरूपदिष्टमार्गेण[6] योगमेव सदाऽभ्यसेत् ॥ 68 ॥

---

1. एकान्तमलिकामध्ये –T,t1. 2. पिटकं –J,n2, गर्त्तपेटकं –N. 3. मण्टप-T.
4. वेदिकोपरिचिरं –T, मण्डपे वेदिकूपरिचिरं –t1. 5. प्राकारसंवेष्टिनं -T.
6. गुरूपदेशमार्गेण-P,T,J.

evaṃvidhe maṭhe sthitvā sarvacintāvivarjitaḥ //
gurūpadiṣṭamārgeṇa yogameva sadā'bhyaset // 68 //

Tr. Staying in such a cottage, one should constantly devote only to the practice of *yoga* as guided by the teacher, giving up all the worries. 68.

त्यक्तनिद्रो मिताहारो[1] जितश्वासो जितेन्द्रियः ॥
हठाभ्यासपरो नित्यं योगी ब्रह्मसमो भवेत् ॥ 69 ॥

tyaktanidro mitāhāro jitaśvāso jitendriyaḥ //
haṭhābhyāsaparo nityaṃ yogī brahmasamo bhavet // 69 //

Tr. A devoted practitioner of *haṭha*, who is consistent in his practice, has gained control over sleep, food, breath and senses, attains *Brahma.* 69.

योगीश्वरस्य योगस्य योगशास्त्रस्य पार्वति ॥
निन्दाञ्च ये प्रकुर्वन्ति राक्षसास्ते नराः[2] क्षितौ ॥ 70 ॥

yogīśvarasya yogasya yogaśāstrasya pārvati //
nindañca ye prakurvanti rākṣasāste narāḥ kṣitau // 70 //

Tr. O *Pārvati* ! One who denounces an adept of *yoga* and science of *yoga*, is like a demon on the earth. 70.

गोधूमशालियवषष्टिकशोभनान्नं[3]
क्षीराज्यमण्ड[4]नवनीतसितामधूनि ॥
शुण्ठीपटोलफलपत्रज[5]पञ्चशाकं
मुद्गादिदिव्यमुदकं च यमीन्द्र[6]पथ्यम् ॥ 71 ॥

godhūmaśāliyavaṣaṣṭikaśobhanānnaṃ
kṣīrājyamaṇḍanavanītasitāmadhūni //
śuṇṭhīpaṭolaphalapatrajapañcaśākaṃ
mudgādidivyamudakaṃ ca yamīndrapathyam // 71 //

Tr. The recommended food items for a *yogī* should comprise good grains like— wheat, rice, barley, *ṣaṣṭika* (a particular variety

---

1. मितहारो -N.2.नरा –P,N. 3.शोभवान्नं -N. 4. मन्द -T.4. शुण्ठीपटौकफलादिक – N,n1,J. 6. यतीन्द्र-N,n1,J.

of rice which takes sixty days to harvest), milk, ghee, cream, butter, sugar candy, honey, dry ginger, *paṭola* fruits (a species of cucumber), the set of five recommended leafy vegetables, green gram and rain water. 71.

Note: The meaning of *maṇḍa* is scum of the boiled rice. The Nepali commentary mentions it as '*motha*', a kind of beans similar to green gram. 71.

कट्वम्लतीक्ष्ण[1]लवणोष्णहरीतशाकं[2]
सौवीरतैलतिलसर्षपमत्स्यमद्यम्[3] ||
अजादि[4]मांसदधितक्रकुलत्थकोद्र-
पिण्याकहिंगुलशुनाद्यमपथ्यमाहुः || 72 ||[5]

kaṭvamlatīkṣṇalavaṇoṣṇaharītaśākam
sauvīratailatilasarṣapamatsyamadyam //
ajādimāṃsadadhitakrakulatthakodra-
piṇyākahiṅgulaśunādyamapathyamāhuḥ // 72 //

Tr. The list of unwholesome food items consists of (tastes like) bitter, sour, pungent, salty, hot, green leafy vegetables, sour gruel, oil, mustard, sesame, fish, alcohol, meat like mutton etc., curd, butter-milk, *kulattha* (a type of lentil), *kodra* (a species of grain), oil-cake, asafoetida, garlic etc. 72.

तथा च[6] गोरक्षवचनम् —
[7]वर्जयेद् दुर्जनप्रीति[8]वह्निस्त्रीपथसेवनम् ||
प्रातःस्नानोपवासादिकायक्लेशादिकं[9] तथा || 73 ||

tathā ca gorakṣavacanam —
varjayeddurjanaprītivahnistrīpathasevanam //
prātaḥsnānopavāsādikāyakleśādikaṃ tathā // 73 //

According to *Gorakṣa*—

Tr. One should shun company of wicked people, fire, women, (long) walk, morning bath, skipping meals and excessive physial strain. 73.

---

1. तिक्त-P. 2. शाक–P,T,t1. 3. 'मपथ्यमाहुः' अधिकपाठः- N. 4. आजादि – P,N,n1. 5. अजादि.......शुनद्यम् — अनुपलब्धः -N. 6. 'च' अनुपलब्धः-P,T,J. 7. तैलाम्ललोणिभीतिभालुकभा- अधिकपाठः-P,T,n2,t1. 8. प्रान्तं-P; प्राप्तं-T,t1. 9. कायक्लेशविधिं -P,T.

मत्स्येन्द्रवचनमपि —
रसमारे मारे हेमकरे मलजारे जारे रोगहरे ॥
वायुपूरे पूरे आयुकरे आत्मध्याने[1] ध्याने मोक्षकरे ॥ 74 ॥
***matsyendravacanamapi* —**
rasamāre māre hemakare malajāre jāre rogahare //
vāyupūre pūre āyukare ātmadhyāne dhyāne mokṣakare //74 //
According to *Matsyendra*—

Tr. Through alchemy of mercury, gold can be produced, purification of the morbidities brings about a disease-free body, longevity can be attained by practice of breathing techniques (*kumbhaka*) and liberation is attained by meditation on the Self. 74.

श्रेष्ठं सुमधुरं स्निग्धं गव्यं धातुप्रपोषणम् ॥
मनोऽभिलषितं योग्यं चतुर्थांशविवर्जितम् ॥
शिवार्पितं च नैवेद्यं योगी भोजनमाचरेत् ॥ 75 ॥
śreṣṭhaṃ sumadhuraṃ snigdhaṃ gavyaṃ dhātupraposạṇam //
mano'bhilaṣitaṃ yogyaṃ caturthāṃśavivarjitam //
śivārpitaṃ ca naivedyaṃ yogī bhojanamācaret // 75 //

Tr. A *yogī* should consume food which is wholesome, sweet, unctuous, containing milk-products, nutritious, food items one relishes, after leaving one-fourth of the stomach empty and after offering of the food to *Śiva*. 75.

अयमेव मिताहारी[2] कदन्नेन[3] विवर्जितः ॥ 76 ॥
ayameva mitāhārī kadannena vivarjitaḥ // 76 //

Tr. A person consuming moderate diet is the one who eschews bad food. 76.

अत्याहारः प्रयासश्च[4] प्रजल्पो नियमग्रहः[5] ॥
जनसंगञ्च लौल्यञ्च षड्भिर्योगो[6] विनश्यति ॥ 77 ॥

---

1. अआघट–N, घटध्याने-J,n1. 2. मितहारी–P. 3. कदन्ने तु-P. 4. प्रवासश्च–N,n1, प्रवाशश्च–J. 5. नियमाग्रहः-N,J. 6. योगी –P.

atyāhāraḥ prayāsaśca prajalpo niyamagrahaḥ //
janasaṅgañca laulyañca ṣaḍbhiryogo vinaśyati // 77 //

Tr. Excess eating, over-exertion, talkativeness, extreme austerity, public contact, and greed— these six ruin *yoga* practice. 77.

उत्साहान्निश्चयाद्[1] धैर्यात्तत्त्वज्ञानार्थदर्शनात्
बिन्दुस्थैर्यान्मिताहाराज्जनसंगविवर्जनात् ॥
निद्रात्यागाज्जितश्वासात् पीठस्थैर्यादनालसात्
गुर्वाचार्यप्रसादाच्च एभिर्योगस्तु[2] सिद्ध्यति ॥ 78 ॥

utsāhānniścayād dhairyāttatvajñānārthadarśanāt
bindusthairyānmitāhārājjanasaṅgavivarjanāt //
nidrātyāgājjitaśvāsāt pīṭhasthairyādanālasāt
gurvācāryaprasādācca ebhiryogastu siddhyati // 78 //

Tr. Success in *yoga* can be attained through these means:— enthusiasm, firm resolution, patience, correct understanding of the principles underlying the phenomenal creation, stability of *bindu*, consumption of moderate food, avoiding public contact and sleep, having control over breath, attaining stability in an *āsana*, diligence, pleasing the *guru* and *ācārya*. 78.

श्रुत्याचार्यप्रसादाच्च योगाभ्यासबलेन च ॥
ईश्वरानुग्रहेणैव[3] योगसिद्धिस्तु[4] जायते ॥ 79 ॥

śrutyācāryaprasādācca yogābhyāsabalena ca //
īśvarānugraheṇaiva yogasiddhistu jāyate // 79 //

Tr. Success in *yoga* can be attained by favour of the (lessons of the) scriptures, grace of *ācārya*, *yoga* practice and grace of *Īśvara*. 79.

श्रीआदिनाथमत्स्येन्द्रशाबरानन्द[5]भैरवाः ॥
शारंगी[6]मीनगोरक्षविरूपाक्षबिलेशयाः ॥ 80 ॥

1. निश्चला-P,T. 2. एभिर्योगश्च-N,J. 3. ईश्वरानुग्रहणेनैव–t1,n4. 4. योगसिद्धिश्च–N,n4,J. 5. सवरानन्द-N, शवरानन्द–n4. 6. सरंगी–N,n1, सारंगी–P, शरंगि-J, सरंगि–n4.

मन्थान[1]भैरवो योगी सिद्धबुद्धिश्च[2] कन्दली ॥
कोरन्दकः[3] सुरानन्दः सिद्धिपादश्च[4] चर्पटी[5] ॥ 81 ॥
करोटिः पूज्यपादश्च नित्यनाथो निरञ्जनः ॥
कपाली[6] बिन्दुनाथश्च काकचण्डीश्वराह्वयः[7] ॥ 82 ॥
अल्लमः प्रभुदेवश्च[8] नैटचूटिश्च[9] टिण्टिणिः[10] ॥
भालुकि[11]र्नागबोधश्च[12] खण्डकापालिकस्तथा[13] ॥ 83 ॥
इत्यादयो महासिद्धाः हठयोगप्रसादतः ॥
खण्डयित्वा कालदण्डं ब्रह्माण्डे विचरन्ति ते ॥ 84 ॥

śrī ādināthamatsyendraśābarānandabhairavāḥ //
śāraṅgī mīnagorakṣavirūpākṣabileśayāḥ // 80 //
manthānabhairavo yogī siddhabuddhiśca kandalī //
korandakaḥ surānandaḥ siddhipādaśca carpaṭī // 81 //
karoṭiḥ pūjyapādaśca nityanātho nirañjanaḥ //
kapālī bindunāthaśca kākacaṇḍīśvarāhvayaḥ // 82 //
allamaḥ prabhudevaśca naiṭacūṭiśca ṭiṇṭiṇiḥ //
bhālukirnāgabodhaśca khaṇḍakāpālikastathā // 83 //
ityādayo mahāsiddhāḥ haṭhayogaprasādataḥ //
khaṇḍayitvā kāladaṇḍaṃ brahmāṇḍe vicaranti te // 84 //

Tr. *Śrī-ādinātha, Matsyendra, Śābara, Ānandabhairava, Śāraṅgī, Mīna, Gorakṣa, Virūpākṣa, Bileśaya, Manthānabhairava, Siddhabuddhi, Kandalī, Korandaka, Surānanda, Siddhipāda, Carpaṭī,*

Karoṭi, Pūjyapāda, Nityanātha, Nirañjana, Kapālī, Bindunātha, Kākacaṇḍīśvara, Allama, Prabhudeva, Naiṭacūṭi, ṭiṇṭiṇi, Bhāluki, Nāgabodha, Khaṇḍakāpālika etc. are the great *siddhas*, who by the power of *haṭha-yoga* defied the whip of *kāla* (death) and freely move in the universe. 80-84.

---

1. मथान-N,n4. 2.सिद्धिबुद्धिश्च-J. 3. गोनन्दक-P,T,J,n1,n4. 4.सिद्धपादश्च–T. 5. पर्पटी–T,t1. 6.कापाली–T, कपालि-n4. 7. काकचण्डश्चरोमकः-J,n1,n4, काकचण्डीश्वरोमयः-T,t1, चण्डीश्वरात्मकः -n2. 8. अल्लमप्रभुदेवश्च-P,T,t1. 9. फैटीछोटी च-P; फैटीछ्रोटी च-T,t1, भैटचूटि च–n4. 10. टिंटिभिः-N,n1,n4, भैवचुटिंटिभिः-J. 11. तालुकिर-P,T,t1. 12. नागलोधश्च–n4. 13. खण्डःकापालिकस्तथा P,T.

Note: Some of the names of *siddhas* seem to have been erroneously written by the scribe. For example, *Kandalī, Korandaka, Karoṭi, Naiṭacūṭi.* It is obvious that these names have been taken from HP(I-5-8). The names of the *siddhas* have different variations in different copies of HP also. However, from the text of HP critically edited by the Lonavla Yoga Institute (India) and on the basis of available information about the names of the *siddhas*, we give below the information available on them.

Ādinātha— A synonym for *Śiva*, who is regarded as the propounder of many *śāstras* including *yoga*. The famous MYS describing *haṭhayoga* is ascribed to *Ādinātha* from whom the *nāthasampradāya* was originated, according to its followers.

Matsyendra—See note on i.3.

Śābara—He was an alchemist and in a text called *śābaratantra*, 12 *kāpālikagurus* renowned for *yoga*, are described.

Ānandabhairava— A *rasasiddha* mentioned in RRS (xvi.7-10). The drugs *ānandabhairavī-vaṭī* and *ānanda-bhairava-rasa* are ascribed to him in RRS.

Śāraṅgī— This seems to be mis-spelt for *cauraṅgī*, a famous disciple of *Matsyendranātha*. A work called *Prāṇasaṅkalī* in Hindī is available on his name. There is also *Cauraṅgīvākyaṃ* on his name, which is included in NP, deposited in RORI, Jodhpur (vide MS No. 16780).

Mīna—There is no agreement about who *Mīnanātha* was. In some traditions *Mīnanātha* is considered as the same as *Matsyendranātha*, but since *Mīna* is separately mentioned here, it seems that he is different from *Matsyendra*. The two works available on his name are *Yogaviṣaya* and *Yogasaṃgraha*.

Gorakṣa— See note on i.3.

Virūpākṣa— On his name three works are available, namely, *Aṣṭasiddhi-vivaraṇaṃ, Amṛtasiddhiyoga* and *Virūpākṣa-pañcāśikā.*

Bileśaya— No information about him is available.

Manthānabhairava— One of the alchemists mentioned in RRS (i.5-7, xii.76-78, xviii.172). The drug *Manthānabhairavarasa* is ascribed to him in RRS (xii.72-74).

Siddhabuddhi— Also described as *Siddhibuddhi.* In some MSS of HP, *siddha* and *buddha* are separately mentioned. In RRS, both *siddha* and *buddha* have been named as alchemists (v.144, xx.107).

Kandalī— Seems wrongly spelt for *Kanthaḍī.* A famous *śaiva-yogī,* who was a contemporary of *Matsyendra* and *Gorakṣa.* He was related to Cola and Cālukya dynasty. His disciples were in Bīḍa region of Mahārāṣṭra. There is *Kanthaḍībodha* on his name deposited in MMPP (1069-70/ 559-60).

Korandaka— Seems to have been wrongly spelt for *Koraṇṭaka.* He is variously referred to as *Karaṇḍaka, Kuraṇṭaka, Pauraṇṭaka* in other MSS of HP. There is a text called *Kapālakuraṇṭaka-haṭhābhyāsapaddhati*, which may be ascribed to him. It describes different *haṭhayogic* practices, especially 112 *āsanas.*

Surānanda— One of the 27 *rasasiddhas* mentioned in RRS (i.225, vi.51-54).

Siddhipāda— He is described as a *rasācārya* in RRS (xvii.120).

Carpaṭi— One of the *rasasiddhas* mentioned in RRS (vi.49-53). *Śrīnivāsa* mentions *Carpaṭi's* view on *jalabasti* (i.50).

He was a contemporary of *Gorakṣa*. King Sāhillavarmā of Cambala Kingdom was his disciple.

Karoṭi— Seems to be mis-spelt for *Kaneri*. He was a disciple of *Nāgārjuna* and residing at Nevāsā in Mahārāṣṭra, which was then the main centre of *raseśvara* tradition. He was residing there between 1078 to 1138 AD and took *samādhi* there around the year 1138 AD.

Pūjyapāda— Probably mis-spelt for *Pūrvapāda*. On his name are found *yoga* and medical treatises such as—*Ratnākarādi-auṣadha-yoga-saṃgraha, Vaidyaka-grantha, Siddhānta-bhāṣya, Nidānamuktāvali* and *Samādhi-śataka.*

Nityanātha— One of the *rasasiddhas* mentioned in PS. He is the author of *Rasaratnākara*. He calls himself *Pārvatī-putra*. According to P. C. Roy, he belongs to about 1300 AD. There is also SSP available on his name. Another work available on his name is *Siddhikhaṇḍa*.

Nirañjana— Mentioned as a *rasasiddha* in PS.

Kapālī— A *rasasiddha* mentioned in RRS (i.2).

Bindunātha—A *rasasiddha*, probably the author of *rasapaddhati*.

Kākacaṇḍīśvara— He was a *rasasiddha* mentioned in the RRS (i.6). There is a published work called *Kākacaṇḍīśvaratantra*. It describes several *kalpas*. Another MS named *Kākacaṇḍeśvaramataṃ* is deposited in the Nepāl Library.

Allamaprabhudeva— He was a contemporary of *Gorakṣa*.

He propounded *Liṅgāyata* cult about 1150 AD. His colleague *Revaṇasiddha* was related to *nāthasaṃpradāya.*

Naiṭa-cūṭi— Seems to have been mis-spelt for *Ghorācoli* or *Ghoḍācoli.* He is also referred to as *Colika* or *Coli.* He was alive in 1266 AD and was staying on *Kiṣkindhā* mountain in Karṇāṭaka. He was a contemporary of *Gorakṣa.* He was more inclined towards *Tantra.* A small treatise called *Ghoḍācolivākyaṃ* is included in NP. There is a drug called *aśvakañcuki* attributerd to him. He is mentioned as a *rasasiddha* in PS.

ṭiṇṭiṇi— A *rasasiddha* mentioned in PS. In some copies of HP, we find the name *Ciñcini.* There is a text called *Ciñcinimatasāra-samuccaya* deposited in Nepāl Library.

Bhāluki— In RRS (ii.143) *Bhāluki* is mentioned as a *rasācārya.*

Nāgabodha— Also called *Nāgabuddhi* mentioned in RRS (i.2-5, vi.49-53, xv.58-65) as an eminent *rasācārya.*

Khaṇḍa— One of the *rasasiddhas* mentioned in the list of 27 *rasācāryas* in RRS (i.5).

Kāpālika— Mentioned as a *rasācārya* in the list of 27 *ācāryas* in RRS (vi.52).

Mahā-siddhas:-

Most of the *siddhas* referred to here are the famous *rasa-siddhas* (alchemists). They were experts in the use of chemical drugs, especially those prepared from mercury, which makes possible the rejuvenation of the body conducive to liberation within the span of life. There is a science called *Raseśvara-darśana* based on the idea of rendering the human body deathless and also the spiritual liberation of man by his nomadic transformation by varied psycho-chemical processes. It is believed that the preservation of the body could be achieved by the use of medicaments. 80-84.

प्राणायामैरेव सर्वे प्रशुष्यन्ति[1] मला इति ॥
आचार्याणान्तु केषाञ्चित् अन्यत्कर्म[2] न सम्मतम्[3] ॥ 85 ॥
prāṇāyāmaireva sarve praśuṣyanti malā iti //
ācāryāṇāntu keṣāñcit anyatkarma na sammatam // 85 //

Tr. *Prāṇāyāma* alone purifies all the morbidities. According to some adepts, no other technique is necessary. 85.

इदं वचनं हठाभ्यासकरणासामर्थ्यमिति[4] बोध्यम्[5] ॥
idaṃ vacanaṃ haṭhābhyāsakaraṇāsāmarthyamiti bodhyam //

Tr. This statement applies to those who are unable to undertake *haṭha* practices.

Note: *Śrīnivāsa* does not agree with the view that *prāṇāyāma* alone removes all kinds of impurities. According to him, efficacy of the purificatory processes cannot be denied. To do so, reflects on the inability of a person to undergo *haṭhayogic* practices.

सम्प्रदायाब्धिमथनाज्जायते रत्नमालिका ॥
सुवर्णखचिता सेयं को वा[6] योगी ह्युपेक्षते[7] ॥ 86 ॥
sampradāyābdhimathanājjāyate ratnamālikā //
suvarṇakhacitā seyaṃ ko vā yogī hyupekṣate // 86 //

Tr. By churning the ocean of different traditions the garland of gems with golden works has been prepared. Which *yogī* would like to ignore this? 86.

---

1. प्रशुध्यन्ते-P,T,t1, प्रशुध्यन्ति-N,n1. 2. अन्यकर्म-N. 3. शंसतं –n4. 4. हठाभ्यासकरणासामर्थ्य-विषयमिति-P,T,t1. 5. बोद्धव्यम् -T,P,t1. 6. सुवर्णखचिता चेत्स्यात्कोवा -P,T,t1. 7. ह्यपेक्षते -T; नुपेक्षते –N,n1, उपेक्षते -J.

Illustrations of Āsanas

Nauli

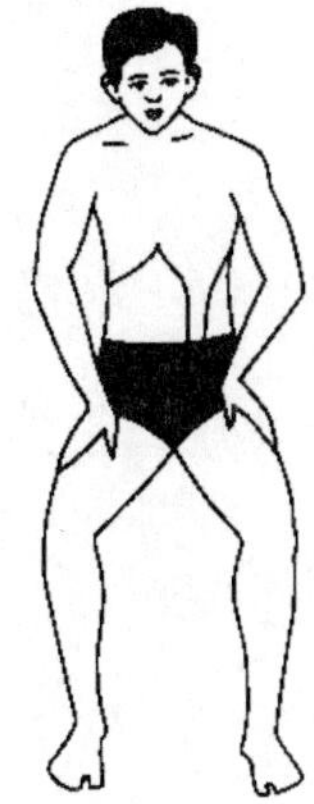

Vāma nauli

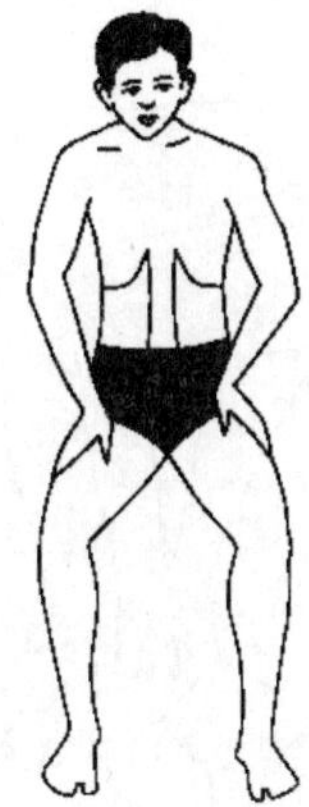

Madhya nauli

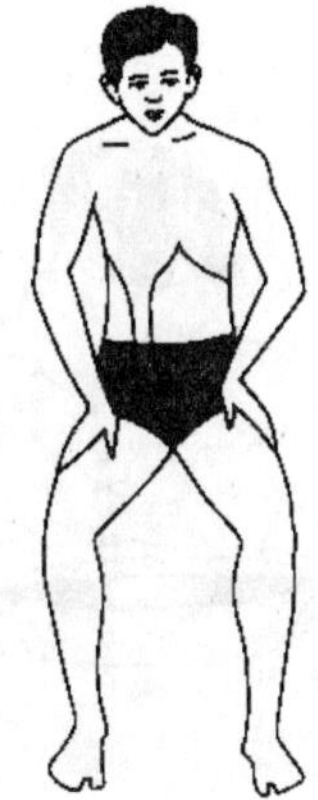

Dakṣiṇa nauli

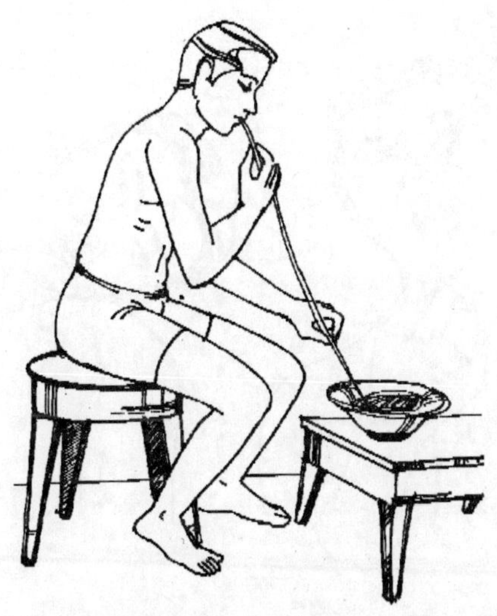

Vastra dhauti

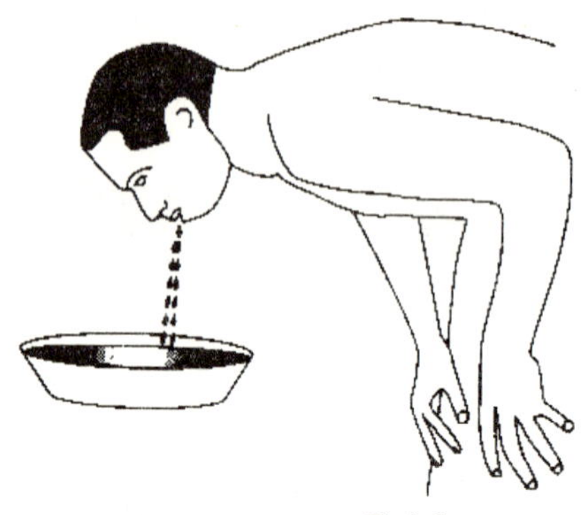

Gajakaraṇī

Sūtra neti

Jalaneti

Illustrations of Āsanas

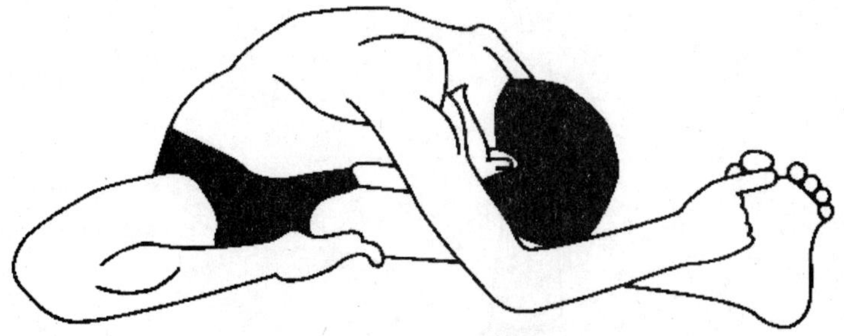

Mahāmudrā

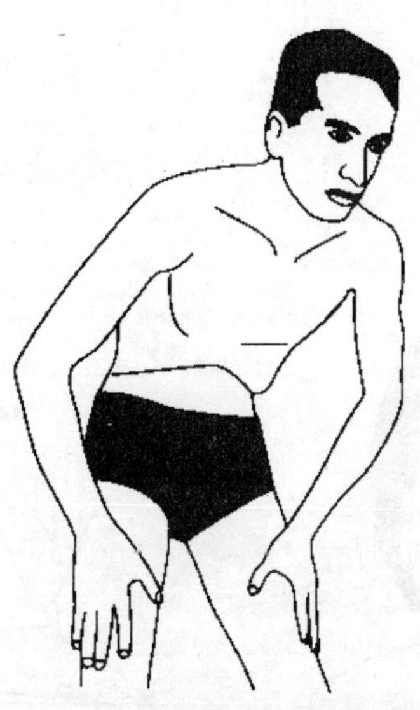

Uḍḍiyāna

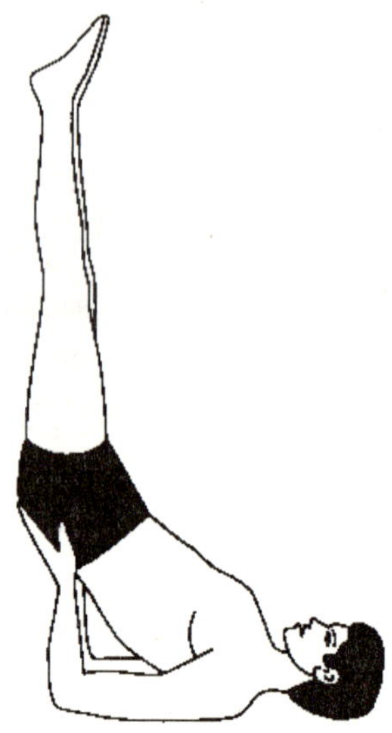

Viparītakaraṇī

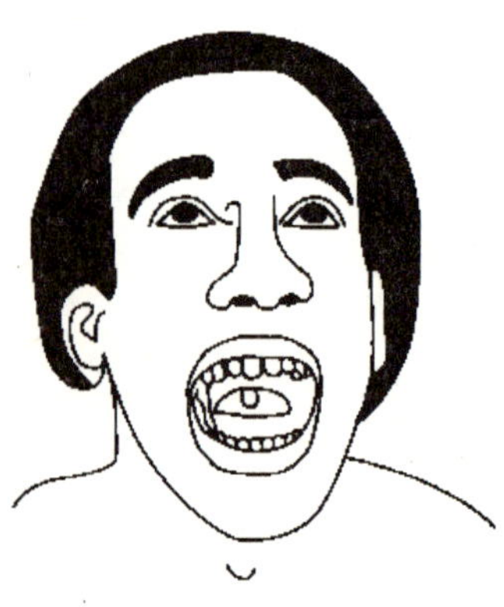

Khecarī

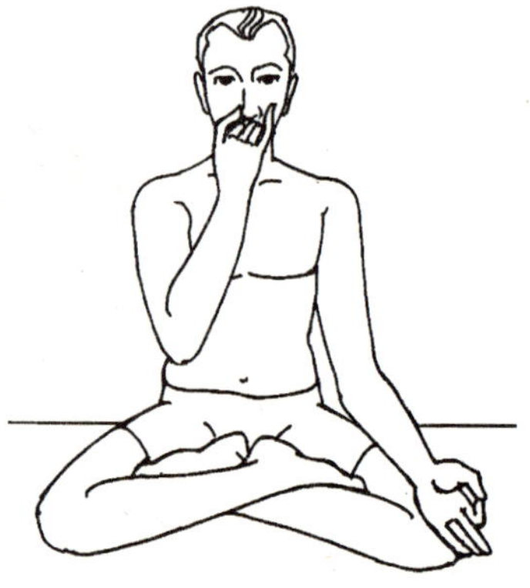

Prāṇāyāma

Note: After this verse, in some MSS, we come across, the qualifications and background of the author, as given in the colophon. 86.

इति श्रीनिवासयोगिविरचितायां[1] हठरत्नावल्यां प्रथमोपदेशः[2].[3]

iti śrīnivāsayogī viracitāyāṃ haṭharatnāvalyāṃ prathamopadeśaḥ

Here ends the first chapter of Haṭharatnāvalī written by Śrīnivāsayogī

---

1. इति श्रीनिवासविरचितायां –J,n2,n4.
2. इति श्रीमत्स्यकलितार्किकचूडामणिसकलन्यायशास्त्रसम्प्रदायप्रवर्तकन्यायाचार्यसकलहठयोगैः प्रवर्तक-तीरभुक्ते देशीयमहादेवमिश्रादिसकलतार्किक्रकवादजयजन्ययशलक्ष्मीविराजगानवैदिकमार्गपतिष्ठैकधुर्यशशधर-मणिकण्ठ-व्याख्यात वेदान्तपरिभाषाद्यनेकग्रन्थकरणजन्यजययशःपुञ्जविद्योतमानतिम्मयज्योतिषिकसोमाम्बात्मज – श्रीनिवासभट्ट- महा -योगीन्द्रविरचितायां हठरत्नावल्यां प्रथमोपदेशः ‖
वेधश्चन्द्रमुखी कराम्बुजलसन्माणिक्यवीणारणत्
तन्त्रे कोमलनाथभंगलहरीमाधुर्यसल्लापिनीम् |
नानार्थांकितचित्रपद्यरचितां वैदग्ध्यविद्योतितां
धत्ते तां हठयोगरत्नसरणीं श्रीश्रीनिवासः स्फुटम् ||P,T,t1. 3. अनुपलब्धपंक्तिः -t1.

हठरत्नावली

द्वितीयोपदेशः[1]

अष्टानां कुम्भकानां तु लक्षणं लक्ष्यते मया[2] ॥
अपूर्वाधिकसिद्ध्यर्थं[3] कुम्भकानभ्यसेत्सुधीः ॥ 1 ॥

aṣṭānāṃ kumbhakānāṃ tu lakṣaṇaṃ lakṣyate mayā //
apūrvādhikasiddhyarthaṃ kumbhakānabhyasetsudhīḥ // 1 //

Tr. The characteristics of eight *kumbhakas* are being narrated by me. A wise should practise the *kumbhakas* to achieve amazing *siddhis*. 1.

अथवा —
विधिवत् प्राणसंयामैः नाडीचक्रे विशोधिते ॥
सुषुम्नावदनं भित्वा सुखाद्विशति[4] मारुतः ॥ 2 ॥[5]

athavā —
vidhivat prāṇasaṃyāmaiḥ nāḍīcakre viśodhite //
suṣumnāvadanaṃ bhitvā sukhādviśati mārutaḥ // 2 //

Or,

Tr. When the group of *nāḍīs* is purified through the prescribed practice of *prāṇāyāma, prāṇa* easily pierces the opening of *suṣumnā* and enters into it. 2.

मारुते मध्यमे जाते[6] मनःस्थैर्यं प्रजायते[7] ॥
मनसः सुस्थिरीभावः सैवावस्था मनोन्मनी ॥ 3 ॥[5]

mārute madhyame jāte manaḥsthairyaṃ prajāyate //
manasaḥ susthirībhāvaḥ saivāvasthā manonmanī // 3 //

Tr. Mind becomes steady as the *prāṇa* moves into the middle path (i.e. *suṣumnā*). This poised state of the mind is called *manonmanī*. 3.

---

1. अथ द्वितीयोपदेशः प्रारभ्यते-R. 2. लक्ष्यतेऽधुना-P,T,t1. 3. आयुष्याधिकसिद्ध्यर्थ-P; आयुषोधिकसिद्ध्यर्थ-T,t1. 4. मुखाद्विशति-J,N,n1,n4. 5. अनुपलब्धश्लोकः -n2. 6. मध्यसंजाते-T,t1. 7. च जायते-T,t1.

तत्सिद्धये विधानज्ञः सदा[1] कुर्वीत कुम्भकान्[2] ॥
विचित्रकुम्भकाभ्यासाद्विचित्रां सिद्धि[3]माप्नुयात् ॥ 4 ॥*
tatsiddhaye vidhānajñaḥ sadā kurvīta kumbhakān //
vicitrakumbhakābhyāsādvicitrāṃ siddhimāpnuyāt // 4 //

Tr. For attaining such a state (of *manonmanī)* the experts practise varieties of *kuṃbhakas.* Amazing results can be achieved by practising various *kumbhakas.* 4.

भस्त्रिका भ्रामरी[4] सूर्यभेदोज्जायी च[5] शीतली ॥
मूर्च्छानामकसीत्कारं[6] केवल[7]श्चाष्टकुम्भकाः ॥
भुजंगकरणी[8] चेति कुम्भका नवसंख्यकाः ॥ 5 ॥*
bhastrikā bhrāmarī sūryabhedojjāyī ca śītalī //
mūrcchānāmakasītkāraṃ kevalaścāṣṭakumbhakāḥ //
bhujaṅgakaraṇī ceti kumbhakā navasaṅkhyakāḥ // 5 //

Tr. *Bhastrikā, bhrāmarī, sūryabheda, ujjāyī, śītalī, mūrcchā, sītkāra* and *kevala* are the eight *kumbhakas. bhujaṅgakaraṇī* is the ninth *kumbhaka.* 5.

अथवा –
सूर्यभेदनमुज्जायी[9] तथा सीत्कारशीतली ॥[10]
भस्त्रिका[11] भ्रामरी[12] मूर्च्छा केवलश्चाष्टकुम्भकाः ॥ 6 ॥[13] *
athavā –
sūryabhedanamujjāyī tathā sītkāraśītalī //
bhastrikā bhrāmarī mūrcchā kevalaścāṣṭakumbhakāḥ // 6 //
Or,

Tr. *Sūryabhedana, ujjāyī, sītkāra, śītalī, bhastrikā, bhrāmarī, mūrcchā* and *kevala* are the eight *kumbhakas.* 6.

---

1 . चित्रकान्-T,t1. 2. कुम्भकाः-T,t1. 3 . बुद्धि–N,n1,J, बुद्धिं–n4. 4 . भ्रामरीं–T, भ्रमरीं -t1. 5 . सूयभेदोझायाति –T,t1. 6 . सीतकारौ–N,n1,n4,J, सीत्कारां–T,t1. 7 . केवला-T; कवल-N. 8. भुजंगकरिणी-T . 9. सूर्यभेदनमनुझया–t1. 10. पंक्तिः अनुपलब्धा–N,n1,J. 11 . भस्त्रिकां–T,t1. 12 . भ्रामरीं –T,t1. 13 . अनुपलब्धश्लोकः–N,n1,J.
* अनुपलब्धश्लोकः-n2,n4.

Note : This is a quotation from HP. While enumerating eight *kumbhakas*, we find in many other copies of HP *plāvinī* included in place of *kevala.* GhS(v.46) omits *sītkārī* and *plāvinī* and substitutes *sahita* and *kevala*. KP describes more than fifty *kumbhakas,* which are not found in any other texts. For details, refer to KP of *Raghuvīra* published by Lonavla Yoga Institute (India). 6.

पूरकान्ते तु कर्तव्यो बन्धो जालन्धराभिधः ||
कुम्भकान्ते रेचकादौ कर्तव्यस्तूड्डियानकः || 7 || [1]

pūrakānte tu kartavyo bandho jālandharābhidhaḥ //
kumbhakānte recakādau kartavyastūḍḍiyānakaḥ // 7 //

Tr. *Jālandhara* should be practised after *pūraka*, while *uḍḍiyāna* should be practised at the end of *kumbhaka*, but before *recaka* starts. 7.

Note : GhS (v.49) has another version for the practice of *uḍḍiyāna*. According to it, *uḍḍiyāna* should be performed after inhalation and before *kumbhaka* begins. 7.

अधस्तात्कुञ्चनेनाशु कण्ठसंकोचने कृते ||
मध्ये[2] पश्चिमतानेन स्यात्प्राणो ब्रह्मनाडिगः || 8 ||[1]
adhastātkuñcanenāśu kaṇṭhasaṅkocane kṛte //
madhye paścimatānena syātprāṇo brahmanāḍigaḥ // 8 //

Tr. By contraction of the anal muscles (*mūlabandha*), by contraction of the throat (*jālandhara bandha*) and by pulling the abdominal wall backwards (*uḍḍiyāna bandha*), the *prāṇa* enters into the *brahma-nāḍī* (*suṣumnā*). 8.

Note: In this verse, the application of *mūlabandha, jālandhara bandha* and *uḍḍiyāna bandha* is suggested. 8.

अपानमूर्ध्वमुत्थाप्य[3] प्राणं[4] कण्ठादधो नयेत् ||
योगी जराविमुक्तः स्यात् षोडशो वयसा[5] भवेत् || 9 ||[1]

---

1. अनुपलब्धश्लोकः -n2. 2. मध्या –N,n1,J. 3. अपानमूर्ध्वमास्थाय -P,T,t1.
4. घ्राणं –J. 5. वयसो –N,n1,n4,J.

apānamūrdhvamutthāpya prāṇaṃ kaṇṭhādadho nayet //
yogī jarāvimuktaḥ syāt ṣoḍaśo vayasā bhavet // 9 //

Tr. One should raise the *apāna* upwards and take the *prāṇa* downwards below the throat (*jālandhara bandha*). This makes the *yogī* free from old age and he becomes as young as of sixteen years. 9.

Note : Here *mūlabandha* and *jālandhara bandha* are indicated. 9.

अथ सूर्यभेदनं नाम कुम्भकः[1]—
दक्षनाड्या[2] समाकृष्य बहिःस्थं[3] पवनं शनैः ॥
यथा लगति कण्ठात्तु[4] हृदयावधि सस्वनम्[5] ॥ 10 ॥*
यथेष्टं कुम्भयेद्वायुं रेचयेदिडया ततः ॥
कपालं शोधनं चापि रेचयेत्पवनं शनैः[6] ॥ 11 ॥ *
आलस्यं वातदोषघ्नं कृमिकीटं निहन्ति च ॥ [7]
पुनः पुनरिदं कार्यं सूर्यभेदाख्यकुम्भकम् ॥ 12 ॥ [8] *

atha sūryabhedanaṃ nāma kumbhakaḥ —
dakṣanāḍyā samākṛṣya bahiḥsthaṃ pavanaṃ śanaiḥ //
yathā lagati kaṇṭhāttu hṛdayāvadhi sasvanam // 10 //
yatheṣṭaṃ kumbhayedvāyuṃ recayediḍayā tataḥ //
kapālaṃ śodhanaṃ cāpi recayetpavanaṃ śanaiḥ // 11 //
ālasyaṃ vātadoṣaghnaṃ kṛmikīṭaṃ nihanti ca //
punaḥ punaridaṃ kāryaṃ sūryabhedākhyakumbhakam //12 //

Tr. Slowly draw the external air through the right nostril in such a manner that the air causes a friction in the throat upto the heart and a sonorous sound is produced. Retain the air in to the capacity and thereafter slowly exhale through the left nostril. This cleanses the frontal sinuses. This further removes lethargy, rheumatism and worms. This *sūryabhedana kumbhaka* should be practised again and again. 10-12.

---

1 . अथसूर्यभेदः-J,N,n1,n4. 2.दक्षनाड्यां–T,t1. 3. बहिस्थं–T,t1,n4. 4 . हृत्कण्ठे–N,n1,n4,J. 5 . सस्वनः-N,n4,J. 6.कपालशोधनं वातदोषघ्नं कृमिनाशनं –N,n1,n4, कृमिनाशकं-J. 7 . अनुपलब्धपंक्तिः-N,n1,n4,J.8.... . सूर्यभेदाख्यं कुंभमभ्यसेत्-N, पुनः पुनरिदं सूर्यभेदनाख्यं कुम्भमभ्यसेत्-J,n1,n4. *अनुपलब्धश्लोकः -n2.

अथोज्जायी[1] —

मुखं संयम्य[2] नाडीभ्यामाकृष्य[3] पवनं शनैः ॥
यथा लगति हृत्कण्ठं[4] हृदयावधि[5] सस्वनः[6] ॥ 13 ॥ *
पूर्ववत्कुम्भयेत्प्राणं रेचयेदिडया ततः ॥
गले श्लेष्महरं[7] प्रोक्तं[8] देहानलविवर्धनम्[9] ॥ 14 ॥ *
नाडीजालोदराधातुगत[10]दोषविनाशनम् ॥
गच्छता तिष्ठता कार्य[11]मुज्जाय्याख्यं हि कुम्भकम् ॥ 15 ॥ *

***athojjāyī*—**

mukhaṃ saṃyamya nāḍībhyāmākṛṣya pavanaṃ śanaiḥ //
yathā lagati hṛtkaṇṭhaṃ hṛdayāvadhi sasvanaḥ // 13 //
pūrvavatkumbhayetprāṇaṃ recayediḍayā tataḥ //
gale śleṣmaharaṃ proktaṃ dehānalavivardhanam // 14 //
nāḍījālodarādhātugatadoṣavināśanam //
gacchatā tiṣṭhatā kāryamujjāyyākhyaṃ hi kumbhakam // 15 //

Tr. Close the mouth. Slowly inhale fully through both the nostrils with a frictional sound felt from the throat upto the chest. Retain the breath in the manner told before and thereafter exhale through the left nostril. This is *ujjāyī kumbhaka*, which cures the phlegmatic disorders of the throat, increases the bodily fire, removes the morbidities of the network of the *nāḍīs*, stomach and the bodily constituents (*dhātus*). This should be practised all the time. 13-15.

Note The term '*gacchatā tiṣṭhatā*' is not to be understood literally as 'while walking and standing', but to be taken to mean 'all the time'. 13-15.

अथ सीत्कारः[12]—

सीत्कां[13] कुर्यात्तथा वक्त्रे[14] घ्राणेनैव[15] विसर्जयेत्[16] ॥
एवमभ्यासयोगेन कामदेवो द्वितीयकः[17] ॥ 16 ॥ *

---

1. अथोज्जायं–T,t1. 2 . सन्नम्य-P,t1. 3 . नासाभ्यामाकृष्य-J,n1,n4, आकर्ष्य—T,t1. 4 . हृत्कण्ठे-N,n1,n4,J; हृत्कण्ठ-T.5 . हृयावधि-N. 6 . संस्थितः-P,T,t1. 7 . गलेश्लेष्मकफहरं-T; गलश्लेदोषहरं-N,n1,n4;गलश्लेष्मदोषहरं-J. 8 . अनुपलब्ध-N,n1,n4,T,t1. 9 . देहामलविवर्धनम्-T,t1. 10 . नाडीजलोदर-धातुगत-J,P; नाडीजलोदरंधातुगत-N,n1,n4. 11 . गच्छन् तिष्ठन् प्रतीकार्य-P,T,t1, गच्छतः-n4. 12 . अथ सीत्काराख्यकुंभकस्वरूपं निरूप्यते-P,T,t1. 13 . सित्कं-T,t1, सित्कं-P.14 . दद्यात् स्वक्रान्ते-P,t1; दद्यात् स्वके क्रान्ते-T. 15 . घ्राणेचैव-P,T,t1. 16 . विजृंभणं -P,T,t1. 17 . कामदेवाद्वितीयकः-N. * अनुपलब्धश्लोकः-n2.

योगिनीचक्रसंसेव्यः[1] सृष्टिसंहारकारकः[2] ॥
न क्षुधा न तृषा निद्रा नैवालस्यं प्रजायते ॥ 17 ॥ *

atha sītkāraḥ —
sītkāṃ kuryāttathā vaktre ghrāṇenaiva visarjjayet //
evamabhyāsayogena kāmadevo dvitīyakaḥ // 16 //
yoginīcakrasaṃsevyaḥ sṛṣṭisaṃhārakārakaḥ //
na kṣudhā na tṛṣā nidrā naivālasyaṃ prajāyate // 17 //

Tr. One should always inhale through the mouth producing the sound '*sīt*', hold the air in and exhale through the nostrils. With this practice, one becomes like a cupid. He is respected by the *yoginī-cakra*, becomes capable to create and destroy and does not suffer from hunger, thirst, sleep and drowsiness. 16-17.

भवेत्स्वच्छन्ददेहस्तु[3] सर्वोपद्रववर्जितः ॥
अनेन विधिना सत्यं[4] योगीन्द्रो भाति भूतले ॥ 18 ॥ *
bhavetsvacchandadehastu sarvopadravavarjitaḥ //
anena vidhinā satyaṃ yogīndro bhāti bhūtale // 18 //

Tr. Moreover, by this practice, an eminent *yogī* becomes physically fit, remains free from all the worldly sufferings and excells in life. 18.

अथ शीतली[5] —
जिह्वया[6] वायुमाकृष्य पूर्ववत्कुम्भकादनु ॥
शनैरशीतिपर्य्यन्तं[7] रेचयेदनिलं सुधीः ॥ 19 ॥ *
atha śītalī—
jihvayā vāyumākṛṣya pūrvavatkumbhakādanu //
śanairaśītiparyyantaṃ recayedanilaṃ sudhīḥ // 19 //

Tr. One draws the air in through the tongue, retains it in the manner told before and thereafter slowly exhales (through the nostrils). This is performed for eighty rounds. 19.

---

1. योगिनीचक्रसाम्राज्यं-P,T,t1, योगिनीचक्रसंसेव्यं–n4. 2. सृष्टिसंहारकारणं-P,T,t1, कारकं–n4. 3. भवेत्स्वच्छन्ददेहः स्यात्-P. भवेत्स्वच्छन्ददेहस्यात् -T,t1. 4. नित्यं-N, यस्तु- J,n1. 5. अथ शीतली लक्ष्यते-P,T, अनुपलब्धपंक्तिः-t1. शीतली-J. 6. इडया-P,T,t1. 7. शनैस्त्वशीतिपर्यन्त–J, शनैस्तु घ्राणरन्ध्राभ्यां सीतिपर्य-न्तं-n4. * अनुपलब्धश्लोकः -n2.

Note: *Śrīnivāsa* has emphasized on practising *śītalīkumbhaka* upto 80 rounds. This is not mentioned specifically with other types of *kumbhakas.* This indicates great importance he attaches to *śītalī.* KP(143) calls it *kākacañcu kumbhaka* and includes *śītalī* and *sītkārī* under it. KP(144) also attaches a great importance to this *kumbhaka.* 19.

गुल्मप्लीहोदरं[1] दोषं[2] ज्वरपित्तक्षुधातृषाः[3] ॥
विषाणि शीतली नाम कुम्भकोऽयं निहन्ति च ॥ 20 ॥

gulmaplīhodaraṃ doṣaṃ jvarapittakṣudhātṛṣāḥ //
viṣāṇi śītalī nāma kumbhako'yaṃ nihanti ca // 20 //

Tr. *Śītalī kumbhaka* removes dropsy, disorders of the spleen, fever, acidity, and toxicity and controls hunger and thirst. 20.

अथ भस्त्रिका—
रेचकः पूरकश्चैव[4] कुम्भकः प्रणवात्मकः[5] ॥
रेचकोऽजस्रनिःश्वासः पूरकस्तन्निरोधकः[6] ॥
समानसंस्थितो योऽसौ[7] कुम्भकः परिकीर्तितः ॥ 21 ॥

atha bhastrikā—
recakaḥ pūrakaścaiva kumbhakaḥ praṇavātmakaḥ //
recako'jasraniḥśvāsaḥ pūrakastannirodhakaḥ //
samānasaṃsthito yo'sau kumbhakaḥ parikīrtitaḥ // 21 //

Tr. *Prāṇāyāma*, which is of the nature of *praṇava*, is three fold, i.e. *recaka, pūraka* and *kumbhaka. Recaka* stands for exhalation to the limit. *Pūraka* means opposite of it, while *kumbhaka* is maintenance of stillness of breath. 21.

यथैव[8] लोहकाराणां भस्त्री[9] वेगेन चाल्यते ॥
तथैव स्वशरीरस्थं चालयेत्पवनं सुधीः ॥ 22 ॥

---

1. गुल्मप्लीहादिकान्-P,T,t1,n2. 2. दोषान्-P,T,t1,n2. 3. तृषा–J,n1, तृषः-T,t1. 4. पूरकं चैव–T. 5. प्राणसंयमः-P,T,t1. 6. पूरकस्तन्निरोधतः-T. 7. समान संस्थिति रूप-P,T,t1. 8. यथैष-P. 9. भस्त्रा-n4.

यथा[1] श्रमो भवेद् देहे तथा[2] सूर्येण[3] पूरयेत् ॥
यथोदरं भवेत्पूर्णं पवनेन तथा लघु ॥ 23 ॥
धारयेन्नासिकां[4] मध्या[5]तर्जनीभ्यां विना दृढम् ॥
कुम्भकं पूर्ववत्कृत्वा रेचयेदिडयानिलम् ॥ 24 ॥

yathaiva lohakārāṇām bhastrī vegena cālyate //
tathaiva svaśarīrastham cālayetpavanam sudhīḥ // 22 //
yathā śramo bhaveddehe tathā sūryeṇa pūrayet //
yathodaram bhavet pūrṇam pavanena tathā laghu //23//
dhārayennāsikām madhyātarjanībhyām vinā dṛḍham //
kumbhakam pūrvavat kṛtvā recayediḍayānilam // 24 //

Tr. A wise should rapidly blow the bodily air like the bellows of an ironsmith until he becomes exhausted. Thereafter, he should slowly inhale through the right nostril so that the cavity fully fills up with air. Now using the fingers other than the middle and the index fingers, he should firmly hold the nose and retain the air as told before and exhale through the left nostril. 22-24.

वातपित्तश्लेष्महरं शरीराग्निविवर्धनम् ॥
ब्रह्मनाडीमुखेसंस्थ[6]कफाद्यर्गल[7]नाशनम् ॥
विशेषेणैव कर्तव्यं भस्त्राख्यं कुम्भकं त्विदम् ॥ 25 ॥

vātapittaśleṣmaharam śarīrāgnivivardhanam //
brahmanāḍīmukhesaṃsthakaphādyargalanāśanam //
viśeṣeṇaiva kartavyam bhastrākhyam kumbhakam tvidam /25/

Tr. This *bhastrā-kumbhaka* cures the disorders caused due to vitiation of *vāta, pitta* and *kapha* humours, stimulates the gastric fire, removes the obstacles like phlegm etc. stuck up at the opening of *brahma-nāḍī* (*suṣumnā*). This practice should be given a special emphasis. 25.

---

1 . यदा -T. 2 . तदा–T,t1,P. 3 . वेगेन –N,n1,n3,n4,J. 4 . धारयेन्नासिका -N,J,T,t1.
5 . मध्ये-N,n1,n3,n4,J,T,t1. 6. संस्थं –P,T,t1,n3. 7 . कफादिगद –N,n3,n4,J.

Note: There are different varieties of *bhastrikā* described in different texts and traditions. Scientific investigation on *bhastrikā prāṇāyāma* indicated that even prolonged practice of 45 minutes does not lead to an increase in the urinary acidity. For details, refer to YM (vol. 1, No. 1, pp. 9-18).

It has been specifically mentioned in the tradition not to use the index and middle fingers for closing the nose during *kumbhaka.* The rationale of it is not clear. This arrangement of fingers is called *omkāra-mudrā.* 21-25.

अथ भ्रामरी[1]—
वेगोद्घोषं पूरकं[2] भृंगनादं भृंगीनादं रेचकं[3] मन्दमन्दम् ॥
योगीन्द्राणां नित्यमभ्यास[4]योगाच्चित्ते जाता काचिदानन्दलीला[5] ॥ 26 ॥

atha bhrāmarī—
vegodghoṣaṃ pūrakaṃ bhṛṅganādaṃ-
bhṛṅgīnādaṃ recakaṃ mandamandam //
yogīndrāṇāṃ nityamabhyāsayogāc -
citte jātā kācidānandalīlā // 26 //

Tr. One inhales forcefully producing a sonorous sound resembling that of a male bee and exhales quite slowly, while making the sound like that of a female bee. This technique, if practised daily, fills the mind of the *yogī* with exceptionally ecstatic feeling. 26.

Note: The humming sound resembling that of a male bee and a female bee during *pūraka* and *recaka* is produced by pronouncing the nasalised sound as in the word *gaṅgā*, accompanied by the vibrations of the soft palate. GhS (v.73-77) gives a different technique of *bhrāmarī*. 26.

---

1. अथ भ्रामरी नाम कुम्भकं निरूप्यते –P,t1; अथ भ्रमरी नाम कुंभकं निरूप्यते-T, भ्रमरी –n3, अथ भ्रमरी –n4. 2. रेचकं -P,T,t1. 3. पूरकं -P,T,t1. 4. एवमभ्यास –P,T,t1. 5. काचिदानन्दमूर्च्छा -N,n1,n2,n3,n4,J,T,t1.

अथ मूर्च्छा[1] —

पूरकान्ते गाढतरं बद्ध्वा[2] जालन्धरं[3] शनैः ॥
रेचयेन्मूर्च्छनाख्योऽयं[4] मनोमूर्च्छा सुखप्रदा ॥ 27 ॥

***atha mūrcchā* —**

pūrakānte gāḍhataraṃ baddhvā jālandharaṃ śanaiḥ //
recayenmūrcchanākhyo'yaṃ manomūrcchā sukhapradā //27 //

Tr. *Jālandhara bandha* (chin lock) should be practised after the *pūraka* and thereafter one should exhale (while maintaining *jālandhara bandha*). This is *mano-mūrcchā*, which is very pleasing. 27.

अथ केवलः[5] —

रेचकं पूरकं मुक्त्वा सुखं[6] यद्वायुधारणम् ॥
प्राणायामोऽयमित्युक्तः स वै[7] केवलकुम्भकः[8] ॥ 28 ॥

***atha kevalaḥ*—**

recakaṃ pūrakaṃ muktvā sukhaṃ yadvāyudhāraṇam //
prāṇāyāmo'yamityuktaḥ sa vai kevalakumbhakaḥ // 28 //

Tr. Retention of breath with great comfort, irrespective of inhalation or exhalation, is called *kevala-kumbhaka* which is real *prāṇāyāma* . 28.

Note: HP(ii.71) classifies *kumbhaka* into *sahita* and *kevala*. The eight varieties of *kumbhaka* described in HP belong to *sahita* category, in which the breath is retained after inhalation and followed by exhalation. *Kevala kumbhaka* is an advanced stage of *sahita kumbhaka* and is attained irrespective of inhalation or exhalation. Thus *sahita* variety is voluntary, whereas *kevala* is involuntary.

In this verse, the *kevala kumbhaka* is included in the nine *kumbhakas* described by *Śrīnivāsa*.

In GhS(v.84-91), the words *kevalī* and *kevala* seem synonymous and it is a voluntary type of *kumbhaka*. Attainment of

---

1. मूर्च्छा–n3. 2 . बन्धो-J,P,n1,n3, बन्धा-n4. 3. जालन्धरः–N,J,t1. 4.मूर्च्छनाख्येयं–P, मूर्च्छनाख्ये च–T, मूर्च्छनाख्ये –t1. 5 . केवलः-J,n3, अथ केवल कुंभकः-P,T. 6 . मुखे-N,n1,n3,n4,J. 7.सर्वैः -n3,n4. 8. केवलकुम्भेण-n4.

kevala stage is an indication of high progress in *yoga*, where the mind gets absorbed completely. 28.

केवले[1] कुम्भके सिद्धे रेचपूरकवर्जिते[2] ॥
न तस्य दुर्लभं किञ्चित्[3] त्रिषु लोकेषु विद्यते ॥ 29 ॥[4]

kevale kumbhake siddhe recapūrakavarjite //
na tasya durlabhaṃ kiñcit triṣu lokeṣu vidyate // 29 //

Tr. For the one who masters the *kevala-kumbhaka* without inhalation or exhalation, nothing remains unachievable for him in the three worlds. 29.

शक्तः केवलकुम्भेन[5] यथेष्टं वायुधारणम्[6] ॥
एतादृशो राजयोगो[7] कथितो नात्र संशयः ॥ 30 ॥

śaktaḥ kevalakumbhena yatheṣṭaṃ vāyudhāraṇam //
etādṛśo rājayogo kathito nātra saṃśayaḥ // 30 //

Tr. Through the technique of *kevala-kumbhaka*, one can easily hold the breath to one's desire. This is undoubtedly *rājayoga*. 30.

अथ भुजंगीकरणम्[8] —
कण्ठेन पूरयेद्वायुं रेचयेत्कण्ठनालतः ॥
भुजंगीकरणं चेति कुम्भकोऽयं नवमः[9] स्मृतः[10] ॥ 31 ॥ [11]

atha bhujaṅgīkaraṇam—
kaṇṭhena pūrayedvāyuṃ recayetkaṇṭhanālataḥ //
bhujaṅgīkaraṇaṃ ceti kumbhako'yaṃ navamaḥ smṛtaḥ //31 //

Tr. Inhale the air through the throat and exhale also through the throat. This is *bhujaṅgī-karaṇa*, the ninth *kumbhaka*. 31.

Note: *Śrīnivāsa* enumerates *bhujaṅgīkaraṇa* as the ninth

1.केवलं–n3. 2.रेचपूरविवर्जिते-P,T,t1, वर्जितः-N,n1. 3.कश्चित्-T. 4. अनुपलब्धश्लोकः -n4. 5.केवले कुंभके-P, शक्तः केवलकुम्भेन–अनुपलब्धः–n4. 6.वायुधारणे-P,T. 7.राजयोगी-P,J,N,n1,n4. 8. अथ भुजंगी–J,N,n1,n2,n3,n4. 9.कुंभको नव-P,T, कुम्भको नवम–t1. 10. कुम्भकोऽयं नव स्मृतः-J,N,n1,n4, 11. इति कुम्भकः-N.

variety of *kumbhaka*. HP(J) calls *sītkārī kumbhaka* as *bhujaṅga-kumbhaka*. HY also refers to *bhujaṅgīkaraṇa*. *Jayatarāma* calls it *bhuyaṅgama* in JP(chapter-v). The technique of *bhujaṅgīkaraṇa* seems to have some similarity with *bhujaṅginī mudrā* described by GhS in (iii.3,69) and *plāvinī kumbhaka* mentioned in HP-ii.70. 31.

महामुद्रा महाबन्धो महावेधस्तृतीयकः ॥
उड्डियानं मूलबन्धो[1] बन्धो जालन्धराभिधः [2] ॥ 32 ॥
करणी विपरीताख्या वज्रोली शक्तिचालनम् ॥
सम्प्रदाया[3] खेचरी सा[4] दश मुद्राः प्रकीर्तिताः ॥ 33 ॥

mahāmudrā mahābandho mahāvedhastṛtīyakaḥ //
uḍḍiyānaṃ mūlabandho bandho jālandharābhidhaḥ /32//
karaṇī viparītākhyā vajrolī śakticālanaṃ //
sampradāyā khecarī sā daśa mudrāḥ prakīrtitāḥ // 33 //

Tr. The well-known ten traditional *mudrās* are: *mahāmudrā, mahābandha, mahāvedha, uḍḍiyāna, mūlabandha, jālandhara, viparītakaraṇī, vajrolī, śakti-cālana* and *khecarī*. 32-33.

Note: Different texts give different number of *mudrās*. GhS (iii.1-3) describes 25 *mudrās*, in which are also included the 10 *mudrās* mentioned here. The nature of the *mudrās* given by GhS is physical at one hand and psychological at the other. JP gives 24 *mudrās* which are different from the list of GhS. These are — *saṃkṣobhaṇī, drāvaṇī, ākarṣaṇī, vaśyā, unmanī, mahāṅkuśā, trikhaṇḍā, virajā, vīparīta-karaṇa, mūlabandha, kāmarāja, uḍḍiyāna, jālandhara, mahāmudrā, mahābandha (pūrṇagirā), mahāvedha, khecarī, varaṇaka, sahajolī, ṣaṇmukhī, cācarī, bhūcarī, agocarī* and *unmanī*.

JP(603)suggests that *mahāmudrā, mahābandha* and *mahāvedha* are to be practised together. The description of *mahābandha* and *mahāvedha* is differently given.

1.महावंधो-N,J. 2. उड्डियानं मूलबन्धो जालन्धराभिधः-T,t1. 3.सन्ति या -P,T,t1. 4.मुद्रा-P,T,t1, अनुपलब्ध –N.

The place of *mahāmudrā* is said to be *yoni-sthāna*, that of *mahābandha* is *kaṇṭha-sthāna* and that of *mahāvedha* is *daśama-sthāna* (*brahma-randhra*). 32-33.

आदिनाथोदिता मुद्रा अष्टैश्वर्यप्रदायकाः[1] ॥
वल्लभाः सर्वसिद्धानां दुर्लभा महतामपि[2] ॥ 34 ॥

ādināthoditā mudrā aṣṭaiśvaryapradāyakāḥ //
vallabhāḥ sarvasiddhānāṃ durlabhā mahatāmapi // 34 //

Tr. These *mudrās*, propagated by *Ādinātha*, bestow upon one the eight supernatural powers and are highly respected by all the *siddhas*, but are difficult to be achieved even by the great. 34.

इति मुद्रा दश प्रोक्ता आदिनाथेन शम्भुना ॥
एकैका तासु मुख्या स्यान्महासिद्धिप्रदायिनी ॥ 35 ॥

iti mudrā daśa proktā ādināthena śambhunā //
ekaikā tāsu mukhyā syānmahāsiddhipradāyinī // 35 //

Tr. This is the set of ten *mudrās* told by *Ādinātha Śambhu*. Each one of them is of great significance, which brings about great *siddhis* (supernatural powers). 35.

अथ महामुद्रा —
महामुद्रां प्रवक्ष्यामि वशिष्ठेनोक्तमादरात् ॥ 36 ॥

atha mahāmudrā—
mahāmudrāṃ pravakṣyāmi vaśiṣṭhenoktamādarāt // 36 //

Tr. With all respect, I now narrate *mahāmudrā*, as told by *Vaśiṣṭha*. 36.

Note : The reference to *Vaśiṣṭha* on *mahāmudrā* is not traceable.

The technique of *mahāmudrā* given here resembles the technique given in ŚS (iv.16-17).

---

1. प्रदायिकाः-P,T,t1. 2. त्रिदशामपि -P,T,t1; मरुतामपि –N,n1.

There are different traditions giving different techniques of *mahāmudrā.* The general technique of *mahāmudrā* consists of the combination of four different practices, namely, *siddhāsana, paścimatāna, kumbhaka* and application of *bandhas.* We find the following variations in different traditions:—

Śivasaṃhitā tradition— It prescribes only *jālandhara-bandha* omitting both *uḍḍiyāna* and *mūla-bandha.* During *jālandharabandha* the *bhrūmadhya-dṛṣṭi* is not required.

Gheraṇḍa saṃhitā tradition— In this tradition, *mūlabandha* and *uḍḍiyāna-bandha* do not form a part of *mahāmudrā* technique. It advises only *jālandhara-bandha* combined with *bhrūmadhya-dṛṣṭi* or gazing in between the eyebrows.

Brahmānanda's tradition— *Brahmānanda*, the commentator of HP, who is trained in a tradition different from that of *Svātmārāma*, differs on two points. He wants big toe and not the foot to be caught hold of in the hooks of the index fingers and not in the finger lock. Secondly, he advises *jihvā-bandha* to be coupled with *kumbhaka* and not three *bandhas.*

Haṭhapradīpikā tradition—The technique described by *Svātmārāma* requires only two *bandhas*, namely *mūlabandha* and *jālandhara-bandha* during the practice of *mahāmudrā.* He omits *uḍḍiyāna-bandha.*

Bālakṛṣṇa's tradition— While commenting upon *mahāmudrā, Bālakṛṣṇa*, the commentator of HP, mentions another variety of the technique in which *mūlabandha* and *jālandhara-bandha* are hinted and the *vāyu* is to be held in the *brahmarandhra.* He suggests that after practising with *candra-nāḍī* (left nostril), it should be repeated with *sūrya-nāḍī* (right nostril).

Mādhavīya tradition— In the *Mādhavīya* tradition mentioned by Swāmī Kuvalyānanda, the extended leg is caught at the foot with finger-lock. Inhalation is done with sound by partial contraction of glottis as in *ujjāyī*. There is simultaneous practice of all the three *bandhas* namely *mūla, uḍḍiyāna* and *jālandhara* during *kumbhaka*.

A comparison of the various techniques prescribed by different traditions noted above will show that the *Mādhavīya* tradition makes the practice of *mahāmudrā* most difficult. However, it is the most perfect of the lot. As a progression based on simple to difficult principle, the sequence of the practice of *mahāmudrā* may be mentioned as follows—1) ŚS tradition, 2) GhS tradition, 3) *Brahmānanda's* tradition, 4) HP tradition, 5) *Bālakṛṣṇa's* tradition and 6) *Mādhavīya* tradition.

For detailed discussion on *mahāmudrā*, refer to YM (V-1:59-76).

In these techniques, the practice of *mahāmudrā* is to be repeated on both the sides – left and right, for equal number of times. This important point has not been mentioned here by *Śrīnivāsa*. 36.

पादमूलेन वामेन योनिं सम्पीड्य दक्षिणम्[1] ॥
पादं प्रसारितं कृत्वा कराभ्यां पूरयेन्मुखम्[2] ॥
कण्ठे बन्धं[3] समारोप्य पूरयेद्वायुमूर्ध्वतः ॥ 37 ॥

pādamūlena vāmena yoniṃ sampīḍya dakṣiṇam //
pādaṃ prasāritaṃ kṛtvā karābhyāṃ pūrayenmukham //
kaṇṭhe bandhaṃ samāropya pūrayedvāyumūrdhvataḥ // 37 //

Tr. Press the perineum with the left heel, extend the right leg and hold it with both the hands, inhale the air and apply *jālandhara bandha* and retain the air in the upper region. 37.

---

1. दक्षिणे-N,J,n1,n4. 2. पूरयेन्मुखे-P,T,t1. 3. वेधं -J.

यथा दण्डाहतः[1] सर्पो दण्डाकारः प्रजायते ॥
ऋज्वीभूता तथा शक्तिः कुण्डली सहजा[2] भवेत् ॥ 38 ॥
yathā daṇḍāhataḥ sarpo daṇḍākāraḥ prajāyate //
ṛjvībhūtā tathā śaktiḥ kuṇḍalī sahajā bhavet // 38 //

Tr. *Kuṇḍalī śakti* becomes straight, just as a snake hit by a stick, becomes straight. 38.

तथा सा[3] मरणावस्था[4] जायते द्विपुटीस्थिता[5] ॥ 39 ॥
tathā sā maraṇāvasthā jāyate dvipuṭīsthitā // 39 //

Tr. This brings about the cessation of the functioning of the two *nāḍīs* (*iḍā* and *piṅgalā*). 39.

न हि पथ्यमपथ्यं वा रसाः सर्वेऽपि नीरसाः ॥
अपि भुक्तं विषं घोरं पीयूषमिव जीर्यते ॥ 40 ॥
na hi pathyamapathyaṃ vā rasāḥ sarve'pi nīrasāḥ //
api bhuktaṃ viṣaṃ ghoraṃ pīyūṣamiva jīryate // 40 //

Tr. For such a person, there is nothing like recommended or prohibited food. All that is tasteless becomes tasty. Even deadliest poison is digested like milk. 40.

क्षयकुष्ठगुदावर्त[6]गुल्माजीर्णपुरोगमाः[7] ॥
दोषाः सर्वे[8] क्षयं यान्ति महामुद्रां तु योऽभ्यसेत्[9] ॥ 41 ॥
kṣayakuṣṭhagudāvartagulmājīrṇapurogamāḥ //
doṣāḥ sarve kṣayaṃ yānti mahāmudrāṃ tu yo'bhyaset // 41 //

Tr. All the ailments like consumption, skin disease, constipation, glandular enlargement, indigestion and many others are cured by the practice of *mahāmudrā*. 41.

कथितेयं महामुद्रा जरामृत्युविनाशिनी ॥
गोपनीया[10] प्रयत्नेन न देया यस्य कस्यचित् ॥ 42 ॥

---

1. दण्डाकृतः-P,t1. 2. सहसा-P,T,n2,t1. 3. तदासौ-N,n1,n3,n4,J. 4. मरणावस्थां–n4. 5. हरते वियदास्थिताम्-N,n1,J, द्विपुटाश्रिता–n2, विपदास्थिताम्-n3,n4. 6. क्षयकुष्ठ उदावर्त-P. 7. गुल्मप्लीहपुरोगमाः-P; गुल्मौ प्लीहपुरोगमाः-T,t1, गुल्मजीर्णपुरोगमाः-J. 8. तस्य दोषां-T; तस्य दोषाः-P,t1. 9. यो न्यसेत्-P,T,t1. 10. गोपनीयं-T,t1.

kathiteyaṃ mahāmudrā jarāmṛtyuvināśinī //
gopanīyā prayatnena na deyā yasya kasyacit // 42 //

Tr. *Mahāmudrā* removes old age and fear from death. Therefore, it should be carefully guarded and should not be imparted to all and sundry. 42.

अथ महाबन्धः[1] —
पार्ष्णिं वामस्य पादस्य योनि[2]स्थाने नियोजयेत् ॥
वामोरूपरि संस्थाप्य दक्षिणं चरणं तथा ॥ 43 ॥ [3]

atha mahābandhaḥ —
parṣṇiṃ vāmasya pādasya yonisthāne niyojayet //
vāmorūpari saṃsthāpya dakṣiṇaṃ caraṇaṃ tathā // 43 //

Tr. Place the left heel at the perineum, and the right foot on the left thigh. 43.

पूरयेन्मुखतो[4] वायुं हृदये चिबुकं दृढम् ॥
निभृत्य योनिमाकुञ्च्य मनो मध्ये नियोजयेत् ॥
रेचयेच्च शनैरेवं महाबन्धोऽयमुच्यते ॥ 44 ॥

pūrayenmukhato vāyuṃ hṛdaye cibukaṃ dṛḍham //
nibhṛtya yonimākuñcya mano madhye niyojayet //
recayecca śanairevaṃ mahābandho'yamucyate // 44 //

Tr. Inhale through the mouth and firmly apply *jālandhara bandha*. Carefully contract the perineum (applying *mūlabandha*) and direct the mind towards the middle path (*suṣumnā*) and slowly exhale. This is *mahābandha*. 44.

---

1. महाबन्धः-n3. 2 योनिं–J.
3. पूरयित्वा मुखं वायुं हृदये चिबुकं तथा ॥
निष्पीड्य योनिमाकुञ्च्य मनो मध्ये नियोजयेत् ॥–अधिकः पाठः-N,n1,n4, पार्ष्णिवामेन योनिमाकुञ्च्य मनोमध्ये नियोजयेत्-n3,n4. 4. पूरितोन्मुखतो–n4, पूरयित्वा मुखं–J.

अयं योगो[1] महाबन्धस्सर्वसिद्धिप्रदायकः[2] ॥
सव्यांगे[3] च समभ्यस्य दक्षिणांगे समभ्यसेत् ॥ 45 ॥

ayaṃ yogo mahābandhassarvasiddhipradāyakaḥ //
savyāṅge ca samabhyasya dakṣiṇāṅge samabhyaset // 45 //

Tr. This technique of *mahābandha* bestows upon one all the *siddhis* (supernatural powers). This should be practised first on the left and then on the right. 45.

अयं च सर्वनाडीनामूर्ध्व[4]गतिविबोधकः ॥
त्रिवेणीसंगमं धत्ते केदारं प्रापयेन्मनः[5] ॥ 46 ॥

ayaṃ ca sarvanāḍīnāmūrdhvagativibodhakaḥ //
triveṇīsaṅgamaṃ dhatte kedāraṃ prāpayenmanaḥ // 46 //

Tr. This promotes all the currents of *nāḍīs* moving in upward direction, brings about the confluence of the three *nāḍīs* (*iḍā, piṅgalā* and *suṣumnā*) and fixes the mind between the eye-brows (*kedāra*). 46.

Note: The expression '*trīveṇī saṅgama*' indicates the confluence of the three rivers, i.e., *Gaṅgā, Yamunā* and *Sarasvatī*. This analogy is implied here in case of confluence of *iḍā, piṅgalā* and *suṣumnā.* The place of confluence here is called *kedāra*, which is the center of the eyebrows. 46.

रूपलावण्यसम्पन्ना यथा स्त्री पुरुषं विना ॥
महामुद्रामहाबन्धौ[6] निष्फलौ[7] वेधवर्जितौ[8] ॥ 47 ॥

rūpalāvaṇyasampannā yathā strī puruṣaṃ vinā //
mahāmudrāmahābandhau niṣphalau vedhavarjitau // 47 //

Tr. Just as a woman with beauty serves no purpose without a man, similarly, *mahāmudrā* and *mahābandha* are futile without the practice of *vedha* (*mahāvedha*). 47.

1.योगी -P,T,t1. 2.महाबंधं सर्वसिद्धिप्रदायकं-P,n2,T,t1. 3.सर्वांगे-T.4.मूर्ध्वं-T,t1. 5.प्रापयेत्पुनः-N,n1,n3. 6. महाबन्धो–P,t1. 7.निष्फला-T,t1, निषरौ–n4. 8.वेधवर्जिता-T,t1.

अथ महावेधः[1]—
महाबन्धस्थितो[2] योगी कृत्वा पूरकमेकधीः[3] ॥
वायूनां गतिमाकृष्य निभृतं कण्ठमुद्रया ॥ 48 ॥

atha mahāvedhaḥ—
mahābandhasthito yogī kṛtvā pūrakamekadhīḥ //
vāyūnāṃ gatimākṛṣya nibhṛtaṃ kaṇṭhamudrayā // 48 //

Tr. Having adopted *mahābandha*, a *yogī* should carefully inhale the air and apply *jālandhara bandha*. 48.

अष्टधा क्रियते चैतत् यामे यामे दिने दिने ॥
पुण्यसंघात[4]सन्धायी[5] पापौघभिदुरः[6] सदा ॥ 49 ॥

aṣṭadhā kriyate caitat yāme yāme dine dine //
puṇyasaṅghātasandhāyī pāpaughabhiduraḥ sadā // 49 //

Tr. If it is practised eight times a day every three hours (*yāma* = 3 hours), it helps accumulating merits and destroys multitude of sins. 49.

सम्यक् श्रद्धावतामेव सुखं प्रथमसाधने ॥
वह्निस्त्रीपथसेवां च प्रथमं परिवर्जयेत्[7] ॥ 50 ॥

samyak śraddhāvatāmeva sukhaṃ prathamasādhane //
vahnistrīpathasevāṃ ca prathamaṃ parivarjayet // 50 //

Tr. Even for those who are devoted should avoid in the beginning contact with fire, woman and taking long walk, which is beneficial. 50.

समहस्तयुगो[8] भूमौ स्फिचौ[9] सन्ताडयेच्छनैः[10] ॥
अयमेव महावेधः सिद्धिदोऽभ्यासतो[11] भवेत् ॥ 51 ॥

samahastayugo bhūmau sphicau santāḍayecchanaiḥ //
ayameva mahāvedhaḥ siddhido'bhyāsato bhavet // 51 //

---

1. अथ महाबन्धः-n2, महावेधः-n3. 2. महावेधस्थितो-J. 3. पूरकमेकधा-N,n1,n3,n4,J. 4. सन्धान-N,J. 5. सन्ध्यायां-N,n1,n4,J. 6. पापौघभिदुरं-P,T,t1. 7. वह्निस्त्रीपथसेवानामादौ वर्जनमादिशेत्-P,T,t1. 8. समहस्तयुगौ–P,T,t1. 9. स्फितौ-T; स्फिजौ-P,t1; स्फिवोति-J. 10. ताडयेच्छनैः-N,J. 11. सिद्धिदोऽभ्यासदो-P, सिद्धिदाभ्यासतो–J.

Tr. Firmly placing the palms on the ground, one carefully strikes the floor with the posteriors. This is *mahāvedha*, which is accomplished by practice. 51.

एतत्त्रयं महागुह्यं जरामृत्युविनाशनम्[1] ॥
वह्निवृद्धिकरं चैव ह्यणिमादिगुणप्रदम् ॥ 52 ॥
etattrayaṃ mahāguhyaṃ jarāmṛtyuvināśanam //
vahnivṛddhikaraṃ caiva hyaṇimādiguṇapradam // 52 //

Tr. This secret triad alleviates old age and fear of death, stimulates gastric fire and offers the supernatural powers like *aṇimā* etc. 52.

अथोड्यानबन्धः[2]**—**
बद्धो[3] येन सुषुम्नायां प्राणस्तूड्डियते यतः ॥
तस्मादुड्डियानाख्योऽयं योगिभिः समुदाहृतः ॥ 53 ॥[4]
***athoḍyānabandhaḥ*—**
baddho yena suṣumnāyāṃ prāṇastūḍḍiyate yataḥ //
tasmāduḍḍiyānākhyo'yaṃ yogibhiḥ samudāhṛtaḥ // 53 //

Tr. The lock confined to *suṣumnā* which causes the *prāṇa* to rise upwards is called *uḍḍiyāna* by the *yogīs*. 53.

उड्डीनं[5] कुरुते यस्मादविश्रान्तं[6] महाखगः ॥
उड्डियानं तदेव स्यात् तत्र बन्धोऽभिधीयते[7] ॥ 54 ॥[8]
uḍḍīnaṃ kurute yasmādaviśrāntaṃ mahākhagaḥ //
uḍḍiyānaṃ tadeva syāt tatra bandho'bhidhīyate // 54 //

Tr. The practice which takes the great bird (*prāṇa*) always moving upwards incessantly, is called *uḍḍiyāna* , which is explained as under. 54.

Note: This verse has been obviously taken from HP (iii.55), where we get the reading '*tatra bandho'bhidhīyate*' instead of '*mūlabandho'bhidhīyate*'. The same reading is found in DBU-76, VU-v.7, which being appropriate, has been accepted here. 54.

---

1. विनाशकम् -n4. 2. अथ उड्डियानबन्धो निरुप्यते-P,T. 3. बद्ध्वा-P,T,t1,J.
4. अनुपलब्धपंक्तिः-P,T,t1. 5. उड्याणं-P,T,t1, उड्डिनं-n4. 6. अविश्रान्तो–T,t1.
7. मूलबन्धोऽभिधीयते –N,J,P,T, तस्मादुड्डियानं बन्धं –n2, उड्डियानबन्धः-n3.
8. अनुपलब्धपंक्तिः-P,T,t1.

उदरे पश्चिमं तानं[1] नाभेरूर्ध्वं च धारयेत् ॥
उड्डियानो ह्यसौ[2] बन्धो मृत्युमातंगकेसरी ॥ 55 ॥
udare paścimaṃ tānaṃ nābherūrdhvaṃ ca dhārayet //
uḍḍiyāno hyasau bandho mṛtyumātaṅgakesarī // 55 //

Tr. Pull the abdominal wall above the navel towards the back. This is *uḍḍiyāna-bandha*, which removes fear of death, like a lion killing an elephant. 55.

गुरुणा सहजं प्रोक्तं वृद्धोऽपि तरुणो भवेत् ॥
बाह्योड्याणं च कुरुते बाह्यालंकारवर्धनम् ॥ 56 ॥[3]
guruṇā sahajaṃ proktaṃ vṛddho'pi taruṇo bhavet //
bāhyoḍyāṇaṃ ca kurute bāhyālaṅkāravardhanam // 56 //

Tr. As a result of diligent practice of *uḍḍiyāna*, as per the instruction of the *guru*, even an old person becomes young. This is called *bāhyoḍyāṇa*, which enhances the external beauty. 56.

नाभेरूर्ध्वमधो वापि तानं कुर्यात् प्रयत्नतः ॥[4]
षण्मासमभ्यसेन्मृत्युं जयत्येव न संशयः ॥ 57 ॥
nābherūrdhvamadho vāpi tānaṃ kuryāt prayatnataḥ //
ṣaṇmāsamabhyasenmṛtyuṃ jayatyeva na saṃśayaḥ // 57 //

Tr. Effortfully contract (the abdomen) above and below the navel. Thus, in six months, one undoubtedly overcomes (premature) death. 57.

Note: *Uḍḍiyāna* is an exercise of the diaphragm and the ribs. It is practised either in sitting or standing positions. There is no mention about the phase of respirations, but the term *'bāhyoḍyāna'* suggests that it is done under exhalatory condition. However, when *uḍḍiyāna* is practised with *prāṇāyāma*, it is done under inhalatory condition. The anatomico-physiological mechanism differs in these two techniques. For detailed scientific investigation on exhalatory type of *uḍḍiyāna*, refer to YM (vol. 1,2,3,6 & 8). 57.

---

1. ताणं–P,t1. 2. ह्ययं -P,T,t1. 3. अन्यश्लोकः उपलब्धः-
उड्डियानं च सहजं गुरुणा कथितं यथा ॥
अभ्यसेत्तदतन्द्रस्तु वृद्धोऽपि तरुणो भवेत् ॥ -J,N,n1,n3,n4. 4. अनुपलब्धपंक्तिः-P,T,t1,n1,n2.

अथ मूलबन्धः —

पार्ष्णिभागेन सम्पीड्य योनिमाकुञ्चयेद् गुदम् ॥
अपानमूर्ध्वमाकुञ्च्य[1] मूलबन्धोऽयमुच्यते[2] ॥ 58 ॥

atha mūlabandhaḥ —

pārṣṇibhāgena sampīḍya yonimākuñcayed gudam //
apānamūrdhvamākuñcya mūlabandho'yamucyate /58/

Tr. Press the perineum with the heel, contract the anal sphincters and pull the *apāna vāyu* upwards. This is *mūlabandha.* 58.

अधोगतिमपानं वै ऊर्ध्वगं[3] कुरुते बलात् ॥
आकुञ्चनेन तं प्राहुर्मूलबन्धं हि योगिनः ॥ 59 ॥[4]

adhogatimapānaṃ vai ūrdhvagaṃ kurute balāt //
ākuñcanena taṃ prāhurmūlabandhaṃ hi yoginaḥ //59//

Tr. *Apāna*, which has a downward movement, is forcefully raised upwards by contraction. *yogīs* call this *mūlabandha*. 59.

गुदं पार्ष्ण्या च सम्पीड्य[5] वायुमाकुञ्चयेद् बलात् ॥
वारं वारं यथा चोर्ध्वं समायाति समीरणः ॥ 60 ॥[6]

gudaṃ pārṣṇyā ca sampīḍya vāyumākuñcayed balāt //
vāraṃ vāraṃ yathā cordhvaṃ samāyāti samīraṇaḥ /60/

Tr. Press the anus with the heel and forcefully contract *apāna vāyu* repeatedly, so that the *vāyu* moves upwards. 60.

प्राणापानौ नादबिन्दू मूलबन्धेन चैकताम् ॥
गतौ तदा योगसिद्धिं[7] प्राप्नोत्येव न संशयः[8] ॥ 61 ॥

prāṇāpānau nādabindū mūlabandhena caikatām //
gatau tadā yogasiddhiṃ prāpnotyeva na saṃśayaḥ /61/

Tr. Thus, with the practice of *mūlabandha, prāṇa* and *apāna, nāda* and *bindu* are united. Then one certainly attains success in *yoga*. 61.

---

1. अपानवृत्तिमाकृष्य-P,T,t1, अपानमूर्ध्वमाकृष्य–J,n4. 2. मूलबन्धोऽयमिष्यते-P,T,t1. 3. मूर्ध्वगं –n4. 4. श्लोकअनुपलब्धः-T,t1. 5. पार्ष्णिना गुदमापीड्य–n3. 6 अनुपलब्धपंक्तिः-P,T,t1. 7. गत्वा योगस्य संसिद्धिं –n4. 8. ततो योगस्य संसिद्धि यच्छतां नात्र संशयः-T, t1,P.

अपानप्राणयोरैक्यं क्षयो मूत्रपुरीषयोः ॥
युवा भवति वृद्धोऽपि सततं मूलबन्धनात् ॥ 62 ॥
apānaprāṇayoraikyaṃ kṣayo mūtrapurīṣayoḥ //
yuvā bhavati vṛddho'pi satataṃ mūlabandhanāt // 62 //

Tr. As a result of consistent practice of *mūlabandha, apāna* and *prāṇa* are unified, urine and faeces are reduced and even an old person becomes young. 62.

अपाने चोर्ध्वगे[1] जाते प्रयाते वह्निमण्डले ॥
तथानलशिखादीप्ति[2]र्वायुना प्रेरिता यथा[3] ॥ 63 ॥[4]
apāne cordhvage jāte prayāte vahnimaṇḍale //
tathānalaśikhādīptirvāyunā preritā yathā // 63 //

Tr. When *apāna* rises up and reaches the region of fire (navel region), the flame of the fire blazes forth, being fanned by *vāyu*. 63.

Note: *Vahnimaṇḍala* refers to the navel region and *analaśikhā* refers to *jaṭharāgni* or gastric fire. 63.

यातायातौ वह्न्यपानौ[5] मूलरूपस्वरूपकौ ॥
तेनाभ्यन्तः प्रदीप्तस्तु ज्वलनो देहजस्तथा ॥ 64 ॥[6]
yātāyātau vahnyapānau mūlarūpasvarūpakau //
tenābhyantaḥ pradīptastu jvalano dehajastathā // 64 //

Tr. Then the fire and *apāna* take their original form, which intensify the bodily fire. 64.

[7]दण्डाहता[8] भुजंगीव निश्चितं[9] ऋजुतामियात्[10] ॥
बिलं प्रविष्टेव[11] ततो[12] ब्रह्मनाड्यन्तरं[13] व्रजेत् ॥
तस्मान्नित्यं[14] मूलबन्धः कर्तव्यो योगिभिः सदा ॥ 65 ॥[15]

---

1. चोर्ध्वगं–P,n1,n2,n4. 2. दीप्ता-P. 3. तथा–N,n1,n2. 4. श्लोकअनुपलब्धः-T,t1. 5. बाह्यपानौ–J,N,n4. 6. श्लोकअनुपलब्धः- T,P,t1. 7. तेन कुण्डलिनी सुप्ता सन्तप्ता सम्प्रबुध्यते–J,N,n1,n2,n3,n4. 8. दण्डाहतो –T,t1. 9. निश्वस्य-T,P,t1. 10. ऋजुतां व्रजेत्-T,P,t1. 11. प्रविश्य -T,P. 12. तत्रैव-T,P. 13. भुजंगी नान्तरं-T,P,t1, ब्रह्मनाड्यन्तरे–n4. 14. तस्मादयं –n3. 15. अनुपलब्धपंक्तिः-T,P,t1.

daṇḍāhatā bhujaṅgīva niścitaṃ ṛjutāmiyāt //
bilaṃ praviṣṭeva tato brahmanāḍyantaraṃ vrajet //
tasmānnityaṃ mūlabandhaḥ kartavyo yogibhiḥ sadā // 65 //

Tr. Thus, *kuṇḍalinī* certainly becomes straight, like a snake beaten by a stick, and enters the *brahmarandhra* (*suṣumnā*). Therefore, the *yogīs* should always practise *mūlabandha*. 65.

Note: These verses give a rationale of arousal of *kuṇḍalinī* by the practice of *mūlabandha*. 64-65.

अथ जालन्धरः[1]—
कण्ठमाकुञ्च्य हृदये स्थापयेच्चिबुकं दृढम्[2] ‖
बन्धो जालन्धराख्योऽयं[3] **जरामृत्युविनाशकः**[4] ‖
बध्नाति हि शिराजालं[5] **नाधो याति नभोजलम्** * ‖ 66 ‖

***atha jālandharaḥ*—**
kaṇṭhamākuñcya hṛdaye sthāpayeccibukaṃ dṛḍham //
bandho jālandharākhyo'yaṃ jarāmṛtyuvināśakaḥ //
badhnāti hi śirājālaṃ nādho yāti nabhojalam // 66 //

Tr. Contract the throat and press the chin against the chest. This is *jālandhara bandha*, which removes old age and premature death. Moreover, it ties up the nervous network, which restricts the downward flow of the nectar oozing from the space. 66.

ततो जालन्धरो बन्धः कण्ठसंकोचने कृते ‖ [6]
न पीयूषं पतत्यग्नौ न च वायुः प्रकुप्यति * ‖ 67 ‖

tato jālandharo bandhaḥ kaṇṭhasaṅkocane kṛte //
na pīyūṣaṃ patatyagnau na ca vāyuḥ prakupyati // 67 //

Tr. *Jālandhara bandha* adopted by contracting the throat does not allow the nectar to fall into the fire and *vāyu* does not go astray. 67.

---

1. अथ जालन्धरबन्धः -n2, जालन्धरबन्धः -n3. 2. स्थापयेद् दृढमिच्छया -P,T,t1. 3. जालन्धरस्त्वेष-P,T,t1, जालन्धराख्यो य–J. 4. विद्यते येन मारुतः-P,T,t1. 5. शिराज्वालं –J, शिरोजालं–n4. 6. बध्नाति .... कृते -अनुपलब्ध-P,T,n2. * अनुपलब्धपंक्तिः -t1.

Note: The word *jāla* refers to the network of the nerves going through the neck into the brain and *dhara* denotes holding back the nectar by working upon the brain. The purpose of *jālandhara* during *prāṇāyāma* is to exercise considerable pressure on the carotid sinus leading to the stimulation of the carotid nerves, which slow down the heart and with constant practice, a trance like condition may supervene. *Jālandhara bandha* is not only practised during *kumbhaka*, but also during *recaka* in *mūrcchā prāṇāyāma*, bringing about stupor. This technique also indicates the principle of *viparītakaraṇī* involved in it. 66-67.

बन्धत्रयमिदं श्रेष्ठं महासिद्धैश्च सेवितम् ||[1]
सर्वेषां योगतन्त्राणां साधनं योगिनो विदुः || 68 || *

bandhatrayamidaṃ śreṣṭhaṃ mahāsiddhaiśca sevitam //
sarveṣāṃ yogatantrāṇāṃ sādhanaṃ yogino viduḥ // 68 //

Tr. The set of three *bandhas* is of great importance in all the *yogīc* treatises and is even practised by the eminent *siddhas*. 68.

अधस्तात्कुञ्चनेनाशु कण्ठसंकोचने कृते ||[2]
मध्ये पश्चिमतानेन स्यात्प्राणो ब्रह्मनाडिगः[3] || 69 || *

adhastātkuñcanenāśu kaṇṭhasaṅkocane kṛte //
madhye paścimatānena syāt prāṇo brahmanāḍigaḥ // 69 //

Tr. Firmly contract the lower region (apply *mūlabandha*), contract the throat (apply *jālandhara bandha*) and retract in the middle (apply *uḍḍiyāna bandha*). Thus, *prāṇa* moves in the *brahmanāḍī*. 69.

Note : This verse indicates the application of three *bandhas*, namely, *mūlabandha*, *jālandhara bandha* and *uḍḍiyāna bandha*, which are practised simultaneously. 69.

---

1. न पीयूषं .... सेवितम् -अनुपलब्धः-P,T. 2. सर्वेषां ....कृते - अनुपलब्धः P,T.
3. मध्ये नाडिगः -n 4. * अनुपलब्धश्लोकः -t1.

मूलस्थानं समाकुञ्च्य उड्डियानं तु कारयेत् ‖ [1]
इडां च पिंगलां बद्ध्वा वाहयेत् पश्चिमं पथम् ‖ 70 ‖[2]

mūlasthānaṃ samākuñcya uḍḍiyānaṃ tu kārayet //
iḍāṃ ca piṅgalāṃ baddhvā vāhayet paścimaṃ patham //70 //

Tr. Adopt *mūlabandha* and practise *uḍḍiyāna*. This closing of *iḍā* and *piṅgalā* directs the *prāṇa* into the posterior path (*suṣumnā*). 70.

अनेनैव विधानेन प्रयाति पवनो लयम् ‖
ततो न जायते मृत्युर्जरारोगादिकं तथा ‖ 71 ‖ [3]

anenaiva vidhānena prayāti pavano layam //
tato na jāyate mṛtyurjarārogādikaṃ tathā // 71 //

Tr. Adherence to such techniques alone merges the *pavana* into the *laya* state, which retards untimely death, diseases and old age etc. 71.

अथ विपरीतकरणी[4] —
यत्किञ्चित् स्रवते चन्द्रादमृतं दिव्यरूपि च[5] ‖
तत्सर्वं ग्रसते सूर्यस्तेन पिण्डं[6] विनाशि च[7] ‖ 72 ‖

atha viparītakaraṇī —
yatkiñcit sravate candrādamṛtaṃ divyarūpi ca //
tatsarvaṃ grasate sūryastena piṇḍaṃ vināśi ca // 72 //

Tr. Whatever divine ambrosia is secreted from the moon, all of that is devoured by the sun. That is why the human body decays. 72.

तत्रास्ति दिव्यं करणं सूर्यस्य मुखबन्धनम् ‖
गुरूपदेशतो ज्ञेयं न तु शास्त्रार्थकोटिभिः[8] ‖ 73 ‖
tatrāsti divyaṃ karaṇaṃ sūryasya mukhabandhanam //
gurūpadeśato jñeyaṃ na tu śāstrārthakoṭibhiḥ // 73 //

---

1. मध्ये ...कारयेत् . . अनुपलब्धः-P,T. 2. अनुपलब्धपंक्तिः-P,T,t1.
3. श्लोकअनुपलब्धः- 'कंठ संकोचनेनैव द्वि नाड्या भवति ध्रुवम् / सर्वेषां योगतन्त्राणां कर्तव्यं च मुहुर्मुहुः // अधिकपाठः-P,T,t1. 4. विपरीतकरणी –n3. 5. दिव्यरूपिणः-P,T,t1.
6. बन्धं-P,T,t1. 7. जरायुतं -P,T,t1, विनश्यति-n3. 8. शास्त्रार्धकोटिभिः-P.

Tr. There is a special way to seal the mouth of the sun, which can only be learnt from a *guru* and not by going through millions of scriptures. 73.

ऊर्ध्वं नाभिरधस्तालुरूर्ध्वं भानुरधः शशी ॥
करणी विपरीताख्या गुरुवाक्येन लभ्यते ॥ 74 ॥[1]
ūrdhvaṃ nābhiradhastālurūrdhvaṃ bhānuradhaḥ śaśī //
karaṇī viparītākhyā guruvākyena labhyate // 74 //

Tr. The technique which puts the navel up and palate down, that is, the sun up and the moon down, is called *viparītakaraṇī,* which can be learnt from a *guru.* 74.

करणी विपरीताख्या सर्वव्याधिविनाशिनी ॥
नित्यमभ्यासयुक्तस्य जठराग्निविवर्धिनी[2] **॥ 75 ॥**[3]
karaṇī viparītākhyā sarvavyādhivināśinī //
nityamabhyāsayuktasya jaṭharāgnivivardhinī // 75 //

Tr. A daily practice of *viparītakaraṇī* alleviates all the diseases and stimulates gastric fire 75.

आहारो बहुलस्तस्य सम्पाद्यः साधकेन[4] **वै**[5] **॥**
अल्पाहारो यदि भवेद्देहमग्निर्दहेत्[6] **क्रमात्**[7] **॥ 76 ॥**[8]
āhāro bahulastasya sampādyaḥ sādhakena vai //
alpāhāro yadi bhaveddehamagnirdahet kramāt // 76 //

Tr. Such a practitioner should consume adequate amount of food or else due to inadequate consumption of food, the body will gradually be consumed by the fire. 76.

अधःशिरश्चोर्ध्वपादौ[9] **क्षणं स्यात्प्रथमे दिने ॥**
क्षणाच्च[10] **किञ्चिदधिकमभ्यसेच्च दिने दिने ॥ 77 ॥**[11]

---

1. पत्रमनुपलब्धम्-N, अनुपलब्धश्लोकः -n3. 2. प्रवर्धिनी-P,T. 3. पत्रमनुपलब्धम् -N. 4. साधकस्य-P,T,t1. 5. च-P,T,t1. 6. भवेदग्निर्देहं दहेत्-P,T. 7. क्षणात्-P,T,t1,n3. 8. पत्रमनुपलब्धम्-N. 9. शिरा ऊर्ध्वपादः-P,T,t1. 10. क्षणाच्चेत्-P,T. 11. पत्रमनुपलब्धम्-N.

adhaḥ śiraścordhvapādau kṣaṇaṃ syāt prathame dine //
kṣaṇācca kiñcidadhikamabhyasecca dine dine // 77 //

Tr. On the first day, one should remain in the topsy-turvy position for a short while. Each day one should maintain the posture longer, increasing the time little by little. 77.

वलितं[1] पलितं चैव षण्मासान्न तु[2] दृश्यते ॥
याममात्रं तु यो नित्यमभ्यसेत् स तु कालजित् ॥ 78 ॥[3]

valitaṃ palitaṃ caiva ṣaṇmāsānna tu dṛśyate //
yāmamātraṃ tu yo nityamabhyaset sa tu kālajit // 78 //

Tr. In six months, grey hair and wrinkles disappear. A daily practice of three hours retards premature death. 78.

स्वस्थं यो वर्तमानोऽपि[4] योगोक्तैर्नियमैर्विना ॥
करणी विपरीताख्या श्रीनिवासेन लक्षिता ॥ 79 ॥[5]

svasthaṃ yo vartamāno"pi yogoktairniyamairvinā //
karaṇī viparītākhyā śrīnivāsena lakṣitā // 79 //

Tr. *Viparītakaraṇī* has been propagated by *Śrīnivāsa*, which can be taken up by the healthy person without adhering to *yogic* injunctions. 79.

Note: *Viparītakaraṇī* is not only a technique, but also an important concept in *haṭhayoga*. This is involved in different *yogic* practices like *jālandhara, khecarī* and *jihvābandha. Pratyāhāra* is considered as *viparītakaraṇī* in GŚ (59), which emphasizes on the reversal process. The rationale of reversal of *sūrya* at the navel and *candra* at the root of the palate, leading to the protection of oozing nectar from the moon, is not yet properly understood in terms of modern concept of anatomy and physiology.

The technique of *viparītakaraṇī* is extended to any pose which has its head down and pelvic region raised up, such

---

1. वली च-P,T,t1. 2. षण्मासोर्ध्वं न-P,T,t1. 3. पत्रमनुपलब्धम्-N. 4. परस्वदेववर्त्तमाने-n1,n2,n3,n4 . 5. पत्रमनुपलब्धम् -N.

as *śīrṣāsana* and *sarvāṇgāsana.* KKHP describes the technique of *viparītakaraṇī* as upside down position of the body in which one is advised to swallow the air by mouth and expel it through the anus. 79.

अथ वज्रोली[1]—
वज्रोलीं कथयिष्यामि गोपितां सर्वयोगिभिः ॥
अतीव तद्रहस्यं हि न देयं[2] **यस्य कस्यचित् ॥ 80 ॥**[3]

***atha vajrolī* —**
vajrolīṃ kathayiṣyāmi gopitāṃ sarvayogibhiḥ //
atīva tadrahasyaṃ hi na deyaṃ yasya kasyacit // 80 //

Tr. I shall explain the technique of *vajrolī,* which has been kept secret by all the *yogīs.* This has to be highly guarded and should not be imparted to anybody. 80.

स्वमानैस्तु[4] **समो यस्मात् तस्यैव कथयेद् ध्रुवम् ॥**
पुत्रस्यापि न दातव्यं[5] **गुरुशिष्यक्रमं विना ॥ 81 ॥**[6]

svamānaistu samo yasmāt tasyaiva kathayed dhruvam //
putrasyāpi na dātavyaṃ guruśiṣyakramaṃ vinā // 81 //

Tr. This should be imparted only to the one who is equally meritorious. Without following the tradition of *guru-śiṣya,* this should not be taught even to the son. 81.

कुण्डलीबोधनं सम्यक् नाडीनां परिशोधनम्[7] **॥**
अपानप्राणयोरैक्यं कार्यं वज्रोलिकर्मणा ॥ 82 ॥

kuṇḍalībodhanaṃ samyak nāḍīnāṃ pariśodhanam //
apānaprāṇayoraikyaṃ kāryaṃ vajrolikarmaṇā // 82 //

Tr. *Vajrolī* awakens *kuṇḍalī,* thoroughly cleanses the *nāḍīs* and unifies *apāna* and *prāṇa.* 82.

---

1. अथ वज्रोलिः सम्प्रदायानुरोधेन लक्ष्यते–P,t1. अथ वज्रोलिः सम्प्रदायानुसारेण लक्ष्यते-T, वज्रोली –n3. 2. देया-P.T,t1,n1,n4. 3. पत्रमनुपलब्धम्-N. 4. स्वप्राणैस्तु-P,T,t1,n3,n4. 5. दातव्या-P,T,t1. 6. पत्रमनुपलब्धम्-N. 7. परशोधनम्-P,T.

अभ्यासस्य क्रमं वक्ष्ये सम्प्रदायानुसारतः ॥
कामिनी[1] वा नरो वाथ वज्रोलीं बुद्धिमान्नयेत्[2] ॥ 83 ॥

abhyāsasya kramaṃ vakṣye sampradāyānusārataḥ //
kāminī vā naro vātha vajrolīṃ buddhimānnayet // 83 //

Tr. I shall explain the order of the practice according to the tradition, which should be followed by a wise, whether young woman or man. 83.

फूत्कारोचितं लिंगं रन्ध्राग्रे[3] बहिः स्थाप्यमेकं लिंगरन्ध्रमध्ये[4] स्थाप्यमपरं[5] मिलित्वा नाल[6]द्वयनिरूपणमादौ क्रियते ॥ तयोर्मध्ये फूत्कारो[7]चितं नालस्वरूपं प्रदर्श्यते ॥

phūtkārocitaṃ liṅgaṃ randhrāgre bahiḥ sthāpyamekaṃ liṅgarandhramadhye sthāpyamaparaṃ militvā nāladvayanirūpaṇamādau kriyate // tayormadhye phūtkārocitaṃ nālasvarūpaṃ pradarśyate //

Tr. One hollow tube should be placed in front of the glans penis and the other one should be inserted in the urethra in such a manner that both the ends of the tube meet. The particulars of the tube suitable for blowing are as follows:

काञ्चनस्य च रूपस्य[8] ताम्रस्याप्यथवाऽयसः ॥
नालं[9] कुर्यात्प्रयत्नेन फुत्कारकरणोचितम्[10] ॥ 84 ॥

kāñcanasya ca rūpasya tāmrasyāpyathavā'yasaḥ //
nālaṃ kuryātprayatnena phutkārakaraṇocitam // 84 //

Tr. A hollow tube of gold, silver, copper or iron should be carefully made suitable for blowing. 84.

विंशत्यंगुलदीर्घमानरुचिरं त्वादौ सुवृत्ताल्पगम्
फूत्कारोचितकालरूपसदृशं[11] नालं हठाभ्यासिभिः ॥
प्रोक्तं तादृशमेव लिंगविवरे यत्नेन संस्थापयेत्
फूत्कारं[12] तदनन्तरं प्रकुरुतां[13] वायुर्यथा सञ्चरेत् ॥ 85 ॥

---

1. कामिनीव–N. 2. बुद्धिमांश्चरेत्–J. 3. पूत्कारोचितलिंगरन्ध्राग्रे–P,T,t1. 4. मध्य–P,T,t1. 5. स्थाप्यमानमपरं–P. 6. नाली–T,t1. 7. पूत्कारो-t1. 8. रौप्यस्य–P, रूप्यस्य–T. 9. नालीं –P,T,t1. 10. पूत्कारकरणोचिताम्-P,T,t1. 11. पूत्कारोचित कोलरूपसदृशं-P,T,t1. 12. पूत्कारं–P,T,t1. 13. प्रकुरुते-P,T,t1.

viṃśatyaṅguladīrghamānaruciraṃ tvādau suvṛttālpagam
phūtkārocitakālarūpasadṛśaṃ nālaṃ haṭhābhyāsibhiḥ //
proktaṃ tādṛśamevaliṅgavivare yatnena saṃsthāpayet
phūtkāraṃ tadanantaraṃ prakurutāṃ vāyuryathā sañcaret/85/

Tr. The *haṭha* practitioners should select the tube which is twenty digits in length, smooth, fine, small and rounded at one end, which is suitable for blowing the air forcibly after the hissing of a cobra. Such a tube should be cautiously inserted into the genital. Then one should blow through the tube so that the air enters in. 85.

हठप्रदीपिकाकारस्तु—
यत्नतः शरनालेन फूत्कारं[1] वज्रकन्धरे ॥
शनैः शनैः प्रकुर्वीत वायुसञ्चारकारणात् ॥ 86 ॥

haṭhapradīpikākārastu—
yatnataḥ śaranālena phūtkāraṃ vajrakandhare //
śanaiḥ śanaiḥ prakurvīta vāyusañcārakāraṇāt // 86 //

According to the author of *Haṭhapradīpikā* —

Tr. One should effortfully and slowly blow through the tube into the urethra so that the air enters in. 86.

हठप्रदीपिकाकारमतं[2] हठयोगाभ्यासे[3]ऽज्ञानविलसितमित्युपेक्षणीयम् ॥
haṭhapradīpikākāramataṃ haṭhayogābhyāse'jñānavila - sitamityupekṣaṇīyam //

Tr. The opinion of the author of *Haṭhapradīpikā* should be discarded like the utterance of an ignorant person.

यदि स्याच्छरनाले[4] हि भृशं वायुर्न सञ्चरेत् ॥
वायुसञ्चारणे त्याज्ये[5] शरनालादिकं[6] मतम् ॥ 87 ॥
yadi syāccharanāle hi bhṛśaṃ vāyur na sañcaret //
vāyusañcāraṇe tyājye śaranālādikaṃ matam // 87 //

---

1. पूत्कारं–P,T,t1. 2. हठप्रदीपिकाकारोक्तमतं–P,T. 3. हठयोगांगाभ्यासे–P. 4. स्याच्छरनालं-P. 5. वायुसञ्चारणात्त्याज्यं-T,t1; वायुसञ्चारणाभ्यासार्थ-N,n1,n2,n3,n4; वायुसञ्चारणाभ्यासे–N,n1,n2,n3,n4,J,T,t1. 6. शरं नालोदितं–P, शरनालोदितं मतं–T,t1.

Tr. Since the passing of air is desirable and if the air does not pass sufficiently through the *śaranāla* (reed stalk), then the use of a reed stalk should be avoided. 87.

Note: The criticism of *Śrīnivāsa* about the ignorance regarding *haṭhayoga* practice of *vajrolī* using *śaranāla* seems to be unwarranted. Although the word *śaranāla* occurs in some of the MSS of HP, there are also other copies in which we find the term *śastanāla*. The term *śastanāla* means appropriate tube, which is accepted also by *Śrīnivāsa*. The main purpose of *śaranāla* is to widen the passage of urethra so that the air blown into it could pass through easily. Although the tubes made up of different metals like gold, silver, copper and iron, as suggested by *Śrīnivāsa*, are convenient for blowing the air through them, for *yogīs* who were living in isolated places, had to depend on the natural sources. The *śaranāla* could be easily available on the banks of the rivers. 87.

लिंगरन्ध्रमध्ये[1] स्थापनीयनालस्वरूपं लिंगरन्ध्रविस्तारार्थं निरूप्यते ॥

liṅgarandhramadhye sthāpanīyanālasvarūpaṃ liṅgarandhra-vistārārthaṃ nirūpyate //

Tr. A tube is inserted in the genital to expand the urethra, details of which are as follows:

तन्तुवत्[2] कनकं नालं[3] नागं[4] ताम्रातिनिर्मलम् ॥
नालद्रव्यमिदं प्रोक्तं श्रीनिवासेन योगिना ॥ 88 ॥

tantuvat kanakaṃ nālaṃ nāgaṃ tāmrātinirmalam //
nāladravyamidaṃ proktaṃ śrīnivāsena yoginā // 88 //

Tr. According to *yogī Śrīnivāsa*, the materials ideally required for the tube should be very fine, the purest form of gold, lead or copper. 88.

---

1. लिंगमध्यरन्ध्रं -J, लिंगरन्ध्रमध्य –P,T,t1,n3,n4. 2. जतुवत्-T,t1,P. 3 . नागं-T,t1,P. 4 . भागं-N,n1

निर्मितं त्रिपलैर्नागैर्द्वादशांगुलदीर्घकम्[1] ॥
छत्राकारं प्रकुर्वीत नालं स्निग्धं सितं मृदु ॥ 89 ॥

nirmitaṃ tripalairnāgairdvādaśāṅguladīrghakam //
chatrākāraṃ prakurvīta nālaṃ snigdhaṃ sitaṃ mṛdu // 89 //

Tr. Make the lead tube weighing three *palas* (about 280 gms), twelve digits in length, shaped like an umbrella, smooth, white and fine. 89.

नियोज्यं[2] लिंगरन्ध्रे च निर्भीतः स्थापयेत् क्षणम् ॥
लिंगस्थैर्यं लिंगदार्ढ्यं बहुवीर्यविवर्धनम्[3] ॥ 90 ॥

niyojyaṃ liṅgarandhre ca nirbhītaḥ sthāpayet kṣaṇam //
liṅgasthairyaṃ liṅgadārḍhyaṃ bahuvīryavivardhanam // 90 //

Tr. Insert the tube in the genital without fear and hold it for a moment. This makes the genital stable, strong and offers increment of semen. 90.

नालं काञ्चननिर्मितं मृदुतरं सांगं च नागैः कृतम् ॥
छत्राकारमतः[4] पलत्रययुतं दैर्घ्यं वितस्तैर्मितम्[5] ॥ 91 ॥

nālaṃ kāñcananirmitaṃ mṛdutaraṃ sāṅgaṃ ca nāgaiḥ kṛtam //
chatrākāramataḥ palatrayayutaṃ dairghyaṃ vitastairmitam // 91 //

Tr. A tube made up of gold should be very smooth and the part made up of lead, shaped like an umbrella, weighing three *palas* (about 280 gms) and 12 digits in length could be there. 91.

नालं तादृशमेव लिंगविवरे यत्नेन संस्थापयेत् ॥ 92 ॥

nālaṃ tādṛśameva liṅgavivare yatnena saṃsthāpayet // 92 //

Tr. Cautiously insert such a tube in the urethra. 92.

विस्तारं[6] तदनन्तरं दृढतरं लिंगं ततो जायते ॥
वायुसञ्चारणे जाते ऊर्ध्वमाकृष्यते बलात् ॥ 93 ॥

---

1. दीर्घितम्-T,t1,P. 2. नियोग्यं-T,t1, नियोज्य–P. 3. बहुवीर्यप्रवर्द्धनम्-J. 4. सर्पाकारमतः-N, छत्राकारमथ-T,t1.; 5. वितस्तेर्मितं –J,P,T. 6. द्विस्तरात् -P, विस्तरात् -T.

vistāraṃ tadanantaraṃ dṛḍhataraṃ liṅgaṃ tato jāyate //
vāyusañcāraṇe jāte ūrdhvamākṛṣyate balāt // 93 //

Tr. This widens the urethra, which makes the penis strong, and the air has a free passage so that one can suck *(rajas)* with force. 93.

नारीं रम्यामधःस्थाप्य रहस्ये तु दिगम्बराम् ॥
स्वयं दिगम्बरो भूत्वा उत्तानायास्तथोपरि[1] ॥
शयित्वा कुम्भकं कृत्वा[2] किञ्चिन्नारी स्वयं च हि[3] ॥ 94 ॥
nārīṃ ramyāmadhaḥsthāpya rahasye tu digambarām //
svayaṃ digambaro bhūtvā uttānāyāstathopari //
śayitvā kumbhakaṃ kṛtvā kiñcinnārī svayaṃ ca hi // 94 //

Tr. In a desolate place, having placed a beautiful naked woman below and oneself also being naked, one lies in prone position. The woman also should practise *kumbhaka* a little. 94.

अन्योऽन्यं गाढमालिंग्य योनौ लिंगं निरोपयेत्[4] ॥
मिथस्त्वधरपानं च कुर्यात् गलरवादिकम्[5] ॥ 95 ॥
anyo'nyaṃ gāḍhamāliṅgya yonau liṅgaṃ niropayet //
mithastvadharapānaṃ ca kuryāt galaravādikam // 95 //

Tr. Both should closely embrace each other and the penis should be penetrated in the vagina. Both should kiss and make whinning sounds. 95.

विलिखेच्च नखेनैव धारयेत्स्वेद[6]सम्भवम् ॥
नार्या[7] भगात् पतदबिन्दुम[8]भ्यासेनोदर्ध्वमाहरेत्[9] ॥ 96 ॥
vilikhecca nakhenaiva dhārayetsvedasambhavam //
nāryā bhagāt patadbindumabhyāsenordhvamāharet // 96 //

Tr. Both should pinch (each other) with nails, hold the perspiration, mastering the technique one should suck the *bindu*

---

1. उत्तानायास्तथायतिः-N,n1,n2,n4,J 2. कुर्यात्-T,t1,P. 3. बहिः-T,N,n1,J. 4. निवेशयेत्-n3. 5. ....रहरदिकम्-J,N,n1,n4. 6. घातयेत् -T,P. 7. नालात् -n4. 8. पतद् बिन्दुर् –T,n1,n2,n3,n4,J. 9. ......नोदर्धमावहेत्-T,n1, नालाद् भगात्यतेद्विंदुरभ्यासेनोर्ध्वमावहेत् -J,N,n3.

back from the vagina and also pull back and preserve one's own *bindu*, which is being secreted. 96.

चलितं च निजं[1] बिन्दुमूर्ध्वमाकृष्य रक्षयेत् ॥
एवं संरक्षयेद् बिन्दुं मृत्युं जयति योगवित् ॥ 97 ॥

calitaṃ ca nijaṃ bindumūrdhvamākṛṣya rakṣayet //
evaṃ saṃrakṣayed binduṃ mṛtyuṃ jayati yogavit // 97 //

Tr. One should suck one's own *bindu* which is flowing and preserve it. Thus, preserving the *bindu*, an adept of *yoga* overcomes untimely death. 97.

मरणं बिन्दुपातेन जीवितं[2] बिन्दुधारणात् ॥
चित्तायत्तं नृणां शुक्रं[3] शुक्रायत्तं च जीवितम् ॥
तस्माच्छुक्रं[4] मनश्चैव[5] रक्षणीयं प्रयत्नतः ॥ 98 ॥

maraṇaṃ bindupātena jīvitaṃ bindudhāraṇāt //
cittāyattaṃ nṛṇāṃ śukraṃ śukrāyattaṃ ca jīvitam //
tasmācchukraṃ manaścaiva rakṣaṇīyaṃ prayatnataḥ // 98//

Tr. Secretion of *bindu* causes death, while preservation brings about longevity. Semen of a human being is under mind's control, while longevity is under the control of semen. Therefore, semen and mind should be carefully controlled. 98.

एवं यो भजते नारी[6] तामेव मनसा स्मरेत्[7] ॥ 99 ॥
evaṃ yo bhajate nārī tāmeva manasā smaret // 99 //

Tr. Such a woman, who is favourable, should be mentally perceived. 99.

सिन्दूरसदृशं योनौ स्त्रीणामास्थायिकं रजः ॥
ऋतुमत्या रजोऽप्येवं रजो बिन्दुं च रक्षयेत् ॥ 100 ॥

---

1. चलितं चलितं-T,P,J,n1,n2,n4, वलितं वलितं -T,P.. 2. जीविते – J. 3. चित्तायत्तं भवेन्नृणां –P,T,t1. 4. तस्माच्छुक्लं -t1. 5. मतश्चैव –J. 6. नारीं –P,T,t1,n2,n4. 7. रमेत् -T,P, स्मरन् -n3.

sindūrasadṛśaṃ yonau strīṇāmāsthāyikaṃ rajaḥ //
ṛtumatyā rajo'pyevaṃ rajo binduṃ ca rakṣayet // 100 //

Tr. *Rajas* (menstrual discharge), which is like red lead, is located in the female genital organ. A menstruating woman should preserve both *rajas* and *bindu.* 100.

ऋतुकाले यथा शुक्रं[1] निर्दोषं योनिसंगतम् ॥
तथा तन्मारुतेनैव स्त्रीरक्तेनैकतामियात्[2] ॥ 101 ॥
ṛtukāle yathā śukraṃ nirdoṣaṃ yonisaṅgatam //
tathā tanmārutenaiva strīraktenaikatāmiyāt // 101 //

Tr. At the time of monthly cycle, the pure semen, which is ejaculated in the vagina, mixes up with woman's menstrual discharge, being moved by *vāyu.* 101.

आयुः कर्म च वित्तं च विद्या चैव चतुष्टयम्[3] ॥
आधानकाले लिखितं[4] गर्भस्थस्यैव देहिनः ॥ 102 ॥
āyuḥ karma ca vittaṃ ca vidyā caiva catuṣṭayam //
ādhānakāle likhitaṃ garbhasthasyaiva dehinaḥ // 102 //

Tr. Span of life, *karma* (profession), wealth and education—these four are destined at the very time of conception. 102.

यावद् यावदयं देहो ध्रियते गर्भशायिनः[5] ॥
तावत्तावदभिव्यक्तिर्लिंगस्यास्य प्रजायते ॥ 103 ॥ *
yāvadyāvadayaṃ deho dhriyate garbhaśāyinaḥ //
tāvattāvadabhivyaktirliṅgasyāsya prajāyate // 103 //

Tr. Whenever a creature takes a (gross) body, the causal body gets manifested. 103.

आयुष्यं वर्धते नित्यं यदि बिन्दुः स्थिरो[6] भवेत् ॥
उत्पत्तिस्थितिसंहारे बिन्दुरेको हि कारणम् ॥ 104 ॥ *

1. शुक्लं-P,t1. 2. स्त्रीरेतेनैकतामियात्-P. 3. विद्या निधनमेव च-J,n1,n2,n3,n4, विद्यां चैव चतुष्टयं–P,T,t1. 4. लिखति-P,T. 5. गर्भशायिना–J,N,n1,n3,n4. 6. बिन्दुस्थिरो–T,n1. * अनुपलब्धश्लोकः -n2.

āyuṣyaṃ vardhate nityaṃ yadi binduḥ sthiro bhavet //
utpattisthitisaṃhāre bindureko hi kāraṇam //104 //

Tr. The span of life becomes prolonged if the *bindu* is stabilized. In all the states of birth, sustenance and death, *bindu* alone is responsible. 104.

ततो भवेद्राजयोगी नान्तरा भवति ध्रुवम् ॥
न चिन्मात्रेण सिद्धिः स्यादभ्यासात् पवनस्य वै[1] ॥ 105 ॥ *

tato bhavedrājayogī nāntarā bhavati dhruvam //
na cinmātreṇa siddhiḥ syādabhyāsāt pavanasya vai // 105 //

Tr. Thus (following this method) alone, one can certainly become a *rājayogī* and not otherwise. Neither the practice of *prāṇāyāma* nor thinking alone brings about quick success. 105.

अभ्यासस्य क्रमं वक्ष्ये नारीणां च शनैः शनैः ॥ 106 ॥ *

abhyāsasya kramaṃ vakṣye nārīṇāṃ ca śanaiḥ śanaiḥ /106/

Tr. The order of the (gradual) practice, even for the woman, is being narrated by me. 106.

लिंगं कराभ्यामाकुञ्च्य मणिं[2] चान्तः[3] प्रवेशयेत् ॥
यावन्मणिप्रवेशः स्यात्तावदभ्यासमाचरेत् ॥
ततः परं समर्था चेदूर्ध्वमाकुञ्चयेद्रजः[4] ॥ 107 ॥ *

liṅgaṃ karābhyāmākuñcya maṇiṃ cāntaḥ praveśayet //
yāvanmaṇipraveśaḥ syāttāvadabhyāsamācaret //
tataḥ paraṃ samarthā cedūrdhvamākuñcayedrajaḥ // 107 //

Tr. She should hold the penis with the hands and insert the glans (penis) in. This should be practised till penetration is perfected. After succeeding in it, one should suck the *rajas*. 107.

तस्याः शरीरे नादस्तु[5] बिन्दुतामेव गच्छति ॥
स बिन्दुस्तद्रजश्चैव एकीकृत्य स्वदेहजौ ॥ 108 ॥ *

---

1. पवनः स्वनैः-P,T,t1. 2. मणि -P,T. 3. वातः-T . 4. ..... समर्थः स्यादूर्ध्व......P,T. 5. अनुपलब्धः–J. * अनुपलब्धश्लोकः -n2.

tasyāḥ śarīre nādastu bindutāmeva gacchati //
sa bindustadrajaścaiva ekīkṛtya svadehajau // 108 //

Tr. In her body, the *nāda* gets transformed into *bindu*, when *bindu* and *rajas* produced in the body become united. 108.

वज्रोल्यभ्यासयोगेन योगसिद्धिः करे स्थिता ॥
अज्ञातयोगशास्त्रेण[1] वज्रोलीं स्त्री तु नाभ्यसेत् ॥ 109 ॥
vajrolyabhyāsayogena yogasiddhiḥ kare sthitā //
ajñātayogaśāstreṇa vajrolīṃ strī tu nābhyaset // 109 //

Tr. With the practice of *vajrolī*, success in *yoga* becomes easy. A woman should not take up the practice of *vajrolī*, if she is not well-versed in the *yogic* techniques. 109.

अयं योगः पुण्यवतां धन्यानां तत्त्वशालिनाम् ॥
निर्मत्सराणां सिध्येत न तु मत्सरशालिनाम् ॥ 110 ॥
ayaṃ yogaḥ puṇyavatāṃ dhanyānāṃ tattvaśālinām /
nirmatsarāṇāṃ sidhyeta na tu matsaraśālinām // 110 //

Tr. Those who are pious, courageous, have gained insight into reality and are free from jealousy, attain success in *yoga*, but not those who are envious. 110.

सर्वेषामेव योगानामयं योगः शुभंकरः ॥
तस्मादयं वरिष्ठोऽसौ भुक्तिमुक्तिफलप्रदः ॥ 111 ॥
sarveṣāmeva yogānāmayaṃ yogaḥ śubhaṅkaraḥ //
tasmādayaṃ variṣṭho'sau bhuktimuktiphalapradaḥ // 111 //

Tr. Among all types of *yoga*, this one is auspicious. This is supreme since it brings success both in material as well as in spiritual realms. 111.

सुगन्धिर्योगिनो[2] देहे जायते बिन्दुधारणात्[3] ॥ 112 ॥
sugandhir yogino dehe jāyate bindudhāraṇāt // 112 //

---

1. अज्ञातयोगशास्त्रस्तु –J. 2. सुगन्धो योगिनो –P. 3. दुग्धधारणात् -T.

Tr. Preservation of *bindu* creates pleasant smell in the body of a *yogī*. 112.

अथ सहजोलिः[1]—
सहजोली चामरोली वज्रोल्या एव भेदतः || 113 ||

***atha sahajoliḥ*—**
sahajolī cāmarolī vajrolyā eva bhedataḥ // 113 //

Tr. *Sahajolī* and *amarolī* are merely the variations of *vajrolī*. 113.

Note: *Bhavadeva* in his YB (vii-292), commenting on *vajrolī, sahajolī* and *amarolī* remarks that *sahajolī, amarolī, vajrolī* comprise a composite process. There is no difference between them. They differ in names. But the function remains the same. When the union of *candra* and *sūrya* takes place in the *yonisthāna*, it is called *amarolī*. When one's *bindu* is held inside with the help of *yonimudrā*, it is termed as *sahajolī*. To suck one's *bindu* and raise it upwards is *vajrolī*. 113.

जले सुभस्म[2] निक्षिप्य दग्धगोमयसम्भवम्[3] ||
वज्रोली मैथुनादूर्ध्वं स्त्रीपुंसोश्चांगलेपनम् || 114 ||

jale subhasma nikṣipya dagdhagomayasaṃbhavam //
vajrolī maithunādūrdhvaṃ strīpuṃsoścāṅgalepanam // 114 //

Tr. Both man and woman should besmear the body with clean ashes of cow-dung mixed up with water after the practice of *vajrolī*. 114.

आसीनयोः सुखेनैव[4] मुक्त[5]व्यापारयोः क्षणम् ||
सहजोलिरियं[6] प्रोक्ता कर्तव्या[7] योगिभिः सदा[8] || 115 ||

āsīnayoḥ sukhenaiva muktavyāpārayoḥ kṣaṇam //
sahajoliriyaṃ proktā kartavyā yogibhiḥ sadā // 115 //

---

1. **सहजोली** –P,T,n2,n3. 2. **जलेषु भस्म**–J,n1,n4. 3. **अनुपलब्धपंक्तिः** –T,t1.
4. **मुखेनैव** -J. 5. **मुक्तः** -n1. 6. **सहजोलिरिति**-n1. 7. **श्रद्धया**-P.T,t1. 8. **तथा** -P,T.

Tr. Thus, one remains in a state of Bliss unmindful of the worldly affairs. This is called *sahajolī,* which should always be practised by the *yogīs*. 115.

अथामरोली[1] —
विहाय नित्यां प्रथमां[2] च धारां
विहाय निःसारतयान्त्यधाराम्[3] ॥
निषेव्यते[4] शीतलमध्यधारां
कापालिकैः खण्डमतैरनर्घ्याम्[5] ॥ 116 ॥

***athāmarolī* —**
vihāya nityāṃ prathamāṃ ca dhārāṃ
vihāya niḥsāratayāntyadhārām //
niṣevyate śītalamadhyadhārāṃ
kāpālikaiḥ khaṇḍamatairanarghyām // 116 //

Tr. The first and the last flow, which is useless, should be avoided and the cool middle flow be consumed. This is highly respected by the *Khaṇḍa Kāpālikas.* 116.

अमरीं यः पिबेन्नित्यं नस्यं कुर्याद्दिने[6] दिने ॥
वज्रोलीमभ्यसेन्नित्यममरोलीति[7] कथ्यते ॥ 117 ॥
amarīṃ yaḥ pibennityaṃ nasyaṃ kuryād dine dine //
vajrolīmabhyasennityamamarolīti kathyate // 117 //

Tr. While undergoing the course of *vajrolī,* when one daily drinks and snuffs *amarī* (urine), it is called *amarolī.* 117.

Note: The description of *vajrolīmudrā* is grossly misunderstood by the masses and uninitiated. This has led to consider *vajrolī* as an obsene practice and in some editions of HP, it is completely omitted.

Although *Śrīnivāsa* has elaborately described *vajrolī,* it is important in this connection to note the remarks of *Bhavadeva Miśra*

---

1. अनुपलब्धः–N,n1,n2,n3,n4,J. 2. पित्तोल्बणत्वात्प्रथमं-P.T,t1. 3. विहारनिःसारतयाल्पधारां – J, निःसरयतां तु धारणं–P,T,t1. 4. निषिंचते-P.T,t1. 5. खंडमतैकमय्यां-P.T,t1, खण्डमतैरनर्घ्या-J. 6. कुर्वन्दिने-P.T. 7. ....मभ्यसेदेवममरोलीति-P.T.

in his YB. He says, "The practice of *bindusiddhi* through *vajrolī* is for the infatuated and ignorant people. For the spiritual knowledge, the behaviour consisting of renouncing all the desires, attachments, and ego consciousness leads to Bliss and Ultimate Peace." 80-117.

अथ शक्तिचालनम् —

पुच्छे[1] प्रगृह्य भुजगीं सुप्तामुद्बोधयेदभीः ॥
निद्रां विहाय सा ऋज्वी ऊर्ध्वमुत्तिष्ठते हठात् ॥ 118 ॥

atha śakticālanam —

pucche pragṛhya bhujagīṃ suptāmudbodhayedabhīḥ //
nidrāṃ vihāya sā ṛjvī ūrdhvamuttiṣṭhate haṭhāt // 118 //

Tr. Just as one catches hold of the sleeping serpent by the tail and pulls it up, similarly, one should awaken the *kuṇḍalī* from its slumber. Then she suddenly rises up. 118.

द्वादशांगुल[2]दैर्घ्यञ्च विस्तृतं[3] च षडंगुलम् ॥
हठज्ञैः मृदुलं प्रोक्तं वेष्टनाम्बरलक्षणम्[4] ॥ 119 ॥

dvādaśāṅgula dairghyañca vistṛtaṃ ca ṣaḍaṅgulam //
haṭhajñaiḥ mṛdulaṃ proktaṃ veṣṭanāmbaralakṣaṇam //119//

Tr. An expert of *haṭha* should cover the tongue with a thin, smooth and clean cloth of twelve digits in length and six digits in width. 119.

विस्तारितेन तां जिह्वां वेष्टयित्वा ततः सुधीः[5] ॥
अङ्गुष्ठतर्जनीभ्यां च[6] हस्ताभ्यां धारयेद् ध्रुवम् ॥
स्वशक्त्या चालयेद्वामे दक्षिणे च पुनः पुनः ॥ 120 ॥

vistāritena tāṃ jihvāṃ veṣṭayitvā tataḥ sudhīḥ //
aṅguṣṭhatarjanībhyāṃ ca hastābhyāṃ dhārayed dhruvam //
svaśaktyā cālayedvāme dakṣiṇe ca punaḥ punaḥ // 120 //

---

1. पुच्छं–P,T,t1,n2. 2. द्वादशांगुलि–P,t1. 3. अन्तरं–P,t1. 4. वेष्टिताम्बरलक्षणम्-J. 5. अनन्तर्रविस्तारितेन ......सुधीः-अनुपलब्धपाठः-N,n1,n2,n3,n4,J,t1. वितस्तिप्रमितं दीर्घ विस्तारे च षडंगुलम् ॥ अधिकः पाठः-P.T,t1. 6. तु–T,t1.

Tr. After spreading and covering the tongue with the cloth, a wise should firmly catch hold of it with thumb and index fingers of both the hands and frequently move it to right and left to the capacity. 120.

मुहूर्तद्वयपर्यन्तं निर्भीत[1]श्चालयेदसौ ॥
ऊर्ध्वमाकृष्यते[2] किञ्चित्सुषुम्णां[3] कुण्डलीगताम्[4] ॥
षण्मासाच्चालनेनैव[5] शक्तिस्तस्योर्ध्वगा[6] भवेत् ॥ 121 ॥
muhūrtadvayaparyantaṃ nirbhītaścālayedasau //
ūrdhvamākṛṣyate kiñcitsuṣumṇāṃ kuṇḍalīgatām //
ṣaṇmāsāccālanenaiva śaktistasyordhvagā bhavet // 121 //

Tr. If one fearlessly undertakes this practice for six hours, *kuṇḍalī* rises a little and enters into *suṣumnā.* A six month's practice alone makes the *śakti* rising upwards. 121.

सूर्येण पूरयेद्वायुं[7] सरस्वत्यास्तु चालयेत्[8] ॥
शब्दगर्भाचालनेन[9] योगी रोगैः प्रमुच्यते ॥ 122 ॥
sūryeṇa pūrayedvāyuṃ sarasvatyāstu cālayet //
śabdagarbhācālanena yogī rogaiḥ pramucyate // 122 //

Tr. One should inhale air through right nostril and activate the *sarasvatī* (*kuṇḍalī*), by manipulation of the tongue. Thus, the *yogī* frees himself from the diseases. 122.

Note: The process of *śakticālana* does not seem to have been clearly described and is mixed with *khecarī.* HP(iii.110-116) suggests different practices like inhalation through the right nostril, pressing of *kanda* and practice of *bhastrā* in the process of *śakticālana.* 122.

येन सञ्चालिता[10] शक्तिः स योगी सिद्धिभाजनः ॥
किमत्र बहुनोक्तेन मृत्युं जयति लीलया ॥ 123 ॥
yena sañcālitā śaktiḥ sa yogī siddhibhājanaḥ //
kimatra bahunoktena mṛtyuṃ jayati līlayā // 123 //

1.विभीत-P.T. 2.ऊर्ध्वमाकृष्य तौ-P.T,t1. 3. सुषुम्नां–T,t1. 4.कुण्डलीगता-P.T,t1. 5.अभ्यासाच्चालनेनैव-N,n1,n2,n3,n4,J. 6.शक्तिःस्यादूर्ध्वगा-P.T. 7. सूर्येणापूरयेद्वायुं–J,N. 8.चालनम्-P.T,t1,n2,n4.J. 9.शब्दगर्भचालनेन–P. 10.संचारिता P.T,t1.

Tr. A *yogī,* who stimulates *śakti* (*kuṇḍalī*), accomplishes supernatural powers (*siddhis*). He easily transcends *kāla* (death). What to speak more ? 123.

सशैलवनधात्र्यास्तु[1] यथाधारोऽहि नायकः[2] ॥
अशेषयोगतन्त्राणां तथाधारो हि कुण्डली ॥ 124 ॥
saśailavanadhātryāstu yathādhāro'hi nāyakaḥ //
aśeṣayogatantrāṇāṃ tathādhāro hi kuṇḍalī // 124 //

Tr. Just as the Lord of serpents is the support of the earth, with all her forests and mountains, similarly, *kuṇḍalinī* forms the very substratum of the entire science of *yoga*. 124.

फणी कुण्डलिनी[3] नागी चक्री[4] वक्री सरस्वती ॥
ललना[5] रसना क्षत्री ललाटी[6] शक्तिः शंखिनी[7] ॥ 125 ॥
रज्वी[8] भुजंगी शेषा च कुण्डली सर्पिणी मणिः ॥
आधारशक्तिः कुटिला[9] कराली[10] प्राणवाहिनी[11] ॥ 126 ॥
अष्टवक्रा[12] षडाधारा व्यापिनी कलनाधरा[13] ॥
कुरीत्येवं[14] च विख्याताः शब्दाः पर्यायवाचकाः ॥ 127 ॥
इति शक्तिचालनम्[15] ॥

phaṇī kuṇḍalinī nāgī cakrī vakrī sarasvatī //
lalanā rasanā kṣatrī lalāṭī śaktiḥ śaṅkhinī // 125 //
rajvī bhujaṅgī śeṣā ca kuṇḍalī sarpiṇī maṇiḥ //
ādhāraśaktiḥ kuṭilā karālī prāṇavāhinī // 126 //
aṣṭavakrā ṣaḍādhārā vyāpinī kalanādharā //
kurītyevaṃ ca vikhyātāḥ śabdāḥ paryāyavācakāḥ // 127 //
iti śakticālanam *//*

Tr. *Phaṇī, kuṇḍalinī, nāgī, cakrī, vakrī, sarasvatī, lalanā,*

---

1. सशैलवनधात्रीणां–P,T,t1. 2. यथाधारः सुराचलः-P.T,t1, कुण्डली–n2. 3. फणी कुण्डलिनी-अनुपलब्ध-N,n1,n3. 4. चक्री-अनुपलब्धः-J,n2. 5. लभना-P,n1,n2,n3, दलना-T,t1. 6. क्षेत्रललाटी-P,T,t1. 7. शंकिणी-P,t1; शंकणी-T. 8. रुजी P; रजी-T,t1. 9. कुंडली-P.T,t1. 10. फनाली–n1,2,3, फलाली –n4. अनुपलब्धः-J. 11. माणवहिनी-J, फणवाहिनी–N. 12. अष्टावक्रा-P.T,t1, अष्टवक्त्रा-J,N. 13. ककनोधरा-P.T, कलनोधरा-t1. 14. कुंतीत्येवं-P.T,t1,J, कुरीत्येवं -J. 15. इति चालन विधिः-N,n1, अनुपलब्धपाठः -n2.

rasanā, kṣatrī, lalāṭī, śakti, śaṅkhinī, rajvī, bhujaṅgī, śeṣā, kuṇḍalī, sarpiṇī, maṇi, ādhāraśakti, kuṭilā, karālī, prāṇavāhinī, aṣṭavakrā, ṣaḍādhārā, vyāpinī, kalanādharā, kurī are the wellknown synonyms of *kuṇḍalinī*. 125-127.

Thus finishes *śakticālanam* .

Note: The synonyms of *kuṇḍalinī* given here are not found in other available texts. 125-127.

अथ खेचरीमुद्रा[1]—

खेचरी चान्तिमा मुद्रा अचिराद् ब्रह्मरन्ध्रगा ॥
सुषुम्णगामृता मूर्ध्वा[2] लम्बिका वाचकाः[3] स्मृताः ॥ 128 ॥

***atha khecarīmudrā* —**

khecarī cāntimā mudrā acirādbrahmarandhragā //
suṣumṇagāmṛtā mūrdhvā lambikā vācakāḥ smṛtāḥ // 128 //

Tr. *Khecarī* forms the ultimate *mudrā*, which quickly makes the *prāṇa* move into *brahmarandhra. Suṣumnagā, amṛtā, mūrdhvā, lambikā* are its synonyms. 128.

न क्रमेण विना शास्त्रं[4] नैव शास्त्रं[5] विना क्रमः ॥
शास्त्रं क्रमयुतं[6] ज्ञात्वा तन्यते[7] श्रीमतां भुवि ॥ 129 ॥

na krameṇa vinā śāstraṃ naiva śāstraṃ vinā kramaḥ //
śāstraṃ kramayutaṃ jñātvā tanyate śrīmatāṃ bhuvi // 129 //

Tr. Without a proper order, there is no science and a science cannot be learnt without an order. By learning the science in proper order, one attains success in life. 129.

जिह्वाकृतिनिभं शस्त्रमल्पं तच्छेदने क्षमम्[8] ॥
स्नुहीपत्रनिभं बल्यं[9] शस्त्रं कुर्याद्विचक्षणः[10] ॥ 130 ॥

1.अथ खेचरी–J,n1,n4, अथ खेचरी महामुद्रा दिङ्मात्रं प्रदर्श्यते–P,T,t1. 2.सुषुम्ना गम्यता मूर्ध्वा-P.T, सुषुम्णागामृतामूर्च्छा–J,N,n3. 3. वाचकः-P,T,t1. 4.शास्त्रा-J. 5. न शास्त्रेण-n3. 6. शास्त्रक्रमयुतं–J,P,T,t1. 7.वर्ण्यते-P.T,t1. 8.शस्त्रमाहोस्विच्छेदने क्षमः-P; शास्त्रं आटे ...स्विच्छेदने क्षमं-T,t1. 9.चाल्यं–P,T,t1. 10. अनुपलब्धपंक्तिः-T.

jihvākṛtinibhaṃ śastramalpaṃ tacchedane kṣamam //
snuhīpatranibhaṃ balyaṃ śastraṃ kuryādvicakṣaṇaḥ // 130//

Tr. A wise person should collect a strong weapon resembling the leaf of milk-hedge, appearing like a tongue, which would be able to cut the tongue very little. 130.

Note: The word *śastra* not only refers to weapon, but also is employed for all the ingredients used during the process of *khecarī*. KKHP refers to various *śastras* with the names given to them according to the ingredients used. For example, black pepper is *sūryaśastra*, rock-salt (*saindhava*) is *candra-śastra*, chebulic myrobalan (*harītakī*) is *dhanvantarī śastra*, spear-headed shape of the weapon is *indra-śastra*, cardamom (*elā*) is *brahma-śastra*, scissors are *caurāsī-śastra*, weapon prepared with sulpher (*gandhaka*) or orpiment (*haritāla*) or vermilion (*hiṅgula*) is *bhavānī-śastra*, extract of white leadwort (*citraka-arka*) is *agni-śastra*. 130.

[1]इडायाः पिङ्गलायाश्च सुषुम्णायाश्च मध्यतः ||
प्रज्ञावताङ्गुलिं दत्वा ग्रन्थिमध्यं[2] समुच्छिनेत् || 131 ||
iḍāyāḥ piṅgalāyāśca suṣumṇāyāśca madhyataḥ //
prajñāvatāṅgulim datvā granthimadhyaṃ samucchinet //131//

Tr. The wise should place a finger at the center of *iḍā, piṅgalā* and *suṣumnā* and cut the center of the knot. 131.

द्विनिष्कं निष्कनिष्कार्द्धं[3] पथ्यानागरसैन्धवान्[4] ||
चूर्णयित्वा तु तच्चूर्णं तेन चूर्णेन घर्षयेत्[5] || 132 ||
dviniṣkaṃ niṣkaniṣkārddhaṃ pathyānāgarasaindhavān //
cūrṇayitvā tu taccūrṇaṃ tena cūrṇena gharṣayct // 132 //

Tr. Take 2 *niṣkas* of *pathyā* (chebulic myrobalan), one *niṣka* of *nāgara* (dried ginger) and half *niṣka* of rock salt and powder them. Rub this powder (on the tongue). 132. (1 *niṣka* = 25gms).

---

1. जिह्वाधो ग्रन्थिमालोक्य तिलमात्रं समुच्छिनेत् -अधिकः पाठः-P,T,t1,n1,n2,n3,n4.
2. ग्रन्थे मध्यं-P.T,t1. 3. निष्कपादार्थ-P,T,t1. 4. पथ्यासागरसैंधवान्-P,T,t1.
5. 'चूर्णयित्वा तु ये चूर्ण तेन चूर्णेन् घर्षयेत्' -P,T,t1; ......धारयेत् -N,n1,n3,n4,J.

पूर्वोक्तेन प्रकारेण शक्तिचालनमाचरेत् ||
गोदोहनं यथा तद्वच्छक्तिचालनमाचरेत्[1] || 133 ||
pūrvoktena prakāreṇa śakticālanamācaret //
godohanaṃ yathā tadvacchakticālanamācaret // 133 //

Tr. Practise *śakticālana* as told before, like one milks a cow.133.

पुनः सप्तदिने प्राप्ते तिलमात्रं समुच्छिनेत् || 134 ||
punaḥ saptadine prāpte tilamātraṃ samucchinet // 134 //

Tr. On the seventh day again cut (the frenum) to the thinness of a sesame. 134.

छेदनादिक्रमेणैव यावद् भ्रूमध्यगा भवेत्[2] ||
तावच्छनैः प्रकर्तव्यं श्रीनिवासस्य भाषणम् || 135 ||
chedanādikrameṇaiva yāvadbhrūmadhyagā bhavet //
tāvacchanaiḥ prakartavyaṃ śrīnivāsasyabhāṣaṇam // 135 //

Tr. One should cautiously follow the processes of *chedana* (cutting) etc., so that the tongue touches the center of the eyebrows. This is told by *Śrīnivāsa.* 135.

अत्रायं हठयोगसम्प्रदायः—

शिशुर्लम्बिकायोगेनातीतानागतं[3] जानाति[4] / गर्भनिःसरणाद् भूमिपाते लम्बिकायोगे[5] जिह्वाबन्धो पातिनी[6] भवति / लम्बिका प्रतिबिम्बत्वेन[7] जिह्वायाम्[8] अधोग्रन्थि[9]-सूक्ष्मरूपतया[10] सर्वेषां नराणां प्रत्यक्षतया अद्यापि दृश्यते || तत्रैव लम्बिका प्रतिबन्धकसूक्ष्मग्रन्थिभेदनं कार्यमिति मम[11] प्रतिभाति ||

***atrāyaṃ haṭhayogasampradāyaḥ* —**

śiśurlambikāyogenātītānāgataṃ jānāti / garbha-niḥsaraṇād-bhūmipāte lambikāyoge jihvābandho pātinī bhavati / lambikā pratibimbatvena jihvāyāṃ adhogranthisūkṣmarūpatayā / sarveṣāṃ narāṇāṃ pratyakṣatayā adyāpi dṛśyate / tatraiva lambikā pratibandhakasūkṣmagranthibhedanaṃ kāryamiti mama pratibhāti/

---

1. तद्वत् जिह्वादोहनमाचरेत्-P,T,t1. 2. भ्रूमध्यभागभवेत्-P,T,t1. 3 . . . नातींतं नागतं-P. 4. योगेनातं ...नाति–T. 5. लम्बिकायोग-P; लम्बिका जिह्वा योगे-T. 6. याति-N,n1,n3,J. 7. प्रतिबिबकत्वेन–P,T,t1. 8. जिह्वाया:-P,T. 9. अत्र ग्रन्थः-P,T, अथोग्रन्थः-n3. 10. सूक्ष्मसूयतमा–J. 11. अनुपलब्धः-N,n3.

According to the tradition of *haṭhayoga*—

Tr. Through *lambikā yoga,* an infant knows the past and the future. On coming out of the womb and taking birth, *lambikā yoga* turns out to be *jihvā-bandha,* which is subtly reflected below the tongue as a knot. This can be verified in all the human beings. I feel that one should pierce the band at this subtle knot which obstructs *laṃbikā.*

परमेश्वरप्रोक्तखेचरीनामपटले तु[1]—
स्नुहीपत्रनिभं[2] **शस्त्रं सुतीक्ष्णं स्निग्धनिर्मलम्** ||
समनायां[3] **तु जिह्वायां**[4] **रोममात्रं समुच्छिनेत्** || 136 ||
***parameśvaraprokta khecarīnāmapaṭale tu* —**
snuhīpatranibhaṃ śastraṃ sutīkṣṇaṃ snigdhanirmalam //
samanāyāṃ tu jihvāyāṃ romamātraṃ samucchinet // 136 //
In *khecarī-paṭala as told by Parameśvara*—

Tr. Get a sharp, clean and smooth weapon of the shape of the leaf of milk-hedge. With this the tongue (frenum) has to be evenly cut to a hair's breadth. 136.

रोममात्रछेदने[5] **न विलम्बेन हि लम्बिका** ||
हृदये[6] **ग्रन्थकाराणामाकूतं**[7] **भणितं**[8] **मया** || 137 ||
romamātrachedane na vilambena hi lambikā //
hṛdaye granthakārāṇāmākūtaṃ bhaṇitaṃ mayā // 137 //

Tr. *Lambikā* (*yoga*) is soon attained if one cuts (the frenum) to a hair's breadth. I have explained what has been left unsolved by the writers in the texts. 137.

दत्तात्रेयस्तु —
कपालकुहरे जिह्वा प्रविष्टा[9] **विपरीतगा** ||
भ्रुवोरन्तर्गता दृष्टिर्मुद्रा भवति खेचरी || 138 ||[10]

---

1. परमेश्वर प्रोक्तं पटले तु-N,n1,n2,J. 2. स्नुहीपत्रनिभे–J, स्नुहिपत्रनिभं–P. 3. समतायास्तु-P,T,t1, समतायान्तु-n1. 4. जिह्वा-P, जिह्वाया-T,t1. 5. रोममात्रभेदेन-P,T,t1, रोममात्रच्छेदनेन-n4. 6. हृदयं –n4. 7. हृदयग्रन्थकारणमत्कृतं-P,T,t1. 8. फणितं-T,t1, कथितं–J. 9. अनुपलब्धः-P. 10. 'कपालकुहरे जिह्वा विपरीता गोरन्तर्गता दृष्टिर्मुद्रा भवति खेचरी-t1.

***dattātreyastu*—**
kapālakuhare jihvā praviṣṭā viparītagā //
bhruvorantargatā dṛṣṭirmudrā bhavati khecarī // 138 //
According to *Dattātreya*—

Tr. Fold the tongue and insert it into the nasopharyngeal cavity and fix the gaze between the eyebrows. This is called *khecarī mudrā*. 138.

न रोगो मरणं तस्य न निद्रा न क्षुधा तृषा ॥
न च मूर्च्छा भवेत्तस्य यो मुद्रां वेत्ति खेचरीम् ॥ 139 ॥[1]
na rogo maraṇaṃ tasya na nidrā na kṣudhā tṛṣā //
na ca mūrcchā bhavettasya yo mudrāṃ vetti khecarīm / 139 /

Tr. One who masters *khecarī mudrā,* does not get affected by diseases, death, sleep, hunger, thirst and stupor. 139.

पीड्यते न स[2] रोगेण[3] लिप्यते न च कर्मणा ॥
बाध्यते[4] न च कालेन यो मुद्रां वेत्ति खेचरीम् ॥ 140 ॥
pīḍyate na sa rogeṇa lipyate na ca karmaṇā //
bādhyate na ca kālena yo mudrāṃ vetti khecarīm // 140 //

Tr. One who attains *khecarī mudrā,* does not suffer from disease, does not get bound by *karma* and is not affected by (untimely) death. 140.

हठप्रदीपिकायाम्[5]—
छेदनचालनदोहैः कलां[6] क्रमेण वर्धयेत्तावत् ॥
यावदियं भ्रूमध्ये स्पृशति[7] तदानीं[8] खेचरीसिद्धिः ॥ 141 ॥
***haṭhapradīpikāyām* —**
chedanacālanadohaiḥ kalāṃ krameṇa vardhayettāvat //
yāvadiyaṃ bhrūmadhye spṛśati tadānīṃ khecarīsiddhiḥ /141/

1. **श्लोकः अनुपलब्धः**-P,T,t1. 2. **च**-P,T,t1. 3. **योगेन**-P,T,t1. 4. **बध्यते**–t1,n4. 5. **हठप्रदीपिकाकारोऽपि**-P,T. 6. **कला**–P. 7. **सा यावत् भ्रूमध्यं स्पृशति**-P; **सा याति यावद् भ्रूमध्यं स्पृशति हि**–T,t1,n2. 8. **तदा**-P,n4.

According to HP—

Tr. The tongue should be gradually lengthened by cutting, moving and milking, till it touches the center of the eyebrows. Then alone *khecarī* is attained. 141.

छेदनस्य प्रकारोक्तेरभावान्मूढता यतः ॥
साधारणोक्त्या[1] दुर्बोधान्नांगीकार्यमिदं मतम् ॥ 142 ॥
chedanasya prakārokterabhāvānmūḍhatā yataḥ //
sādhāraṇoktyā durbodhānnāṅgīkāryamidaṃ matam // 142 //

Tr. The opinion given above is unacceptable as it does not provide details, which may lead to confusion of a layman. 142.

गुरुदर्शितमार्गेण संकेतः कथ्यते मया ॥
संकेतशृंखलाभावे खेचरी तु कथं भवेत् ॥ 143 ॥
gurudarśitamārgeṇa saṅketaḥ kathyate mayā //
saṅketaśṛṅkhalābhāve khecarī tu kathaṃ bhavet // 143 //

Tr. I am explaining *saṅketa* as per the guidelines of *guru*. How *khecarī* can be attained without *saṅketa* and *śṛṅkhalā* ? 143.

सर्पाकारं सवलयं शृंखलाद्वयसेवितम्[2] ॥
सखर्परं[3] षड्वितस्तिदैर्घ्यं संकेतलक्षणम् ॥ 144 ॥
sarpākāraṃ savalayaṃ śṛṅkhalādvayasevitam //
sakharparaṃ ṣaḍvitastidairghyaṃ saṅketalakṣaṇam // 144 //

Tr. The characteristics of a *saṅketa* are: shaped like a snake, rounded, containing two *śṛṅkhalās* (chains?), (providing) a skull, measuring six *vitastis* (72 digits) in length. 144.

Note: *Śrīnivāsa* gives here the technique and use of *saṅketa* according to the tradition of his *guru*. The characteristics of *saṅketa* are not found described in the available texts of *yoga*. Although *Śrīnivāsa* describes '*saṅketa*' in the form of two spiral rings for the insertion of the tongue into it, the description is not clear. 144.

---

1. साधारकृणोक्त -P; साधारणोक्ति-T,t1. 2. श्रृंखलाद्वयसंमितं-P,T,t1. 3. सकूर्परं-P,T,t1.

शृंखलाद्वितयनिर्मितां परां[1]
सर्पवद्वलयखर्परान्विताम् ॥
विंशदंगुलमितां सुदीर्घिकां
लम्बिकाभ्युदयकारिणीं[2] विदुः ॥ 145 ॥[3]

śṛṅkhalādvitayanirmitāṃ parāṃ
sarpavadvalayakharparānvitām //
viṃśadaṅgulamitāṃ sudīrghikāṃ
lambikābhyudayakāriṇīṃ viduḥ // 145 //

Tr. (A *saṅketa* is) finely made up of two *śṛṅkhalās,* rounded like a snake, containing *kharpara* (a skull), measuring twenty digits in length, which brings success in *lambikā.* 145.

शृंखलायाश्च वलये जिह्वां तत्र प्रवेशयेत् ॥[4]
यथा भवेत्सुषुम्णागा[5] तथा भवति खेचरी ॥ 146 ॥

śṛṅkhalāyāśca valaye jihvāṃ tatra praveśayet //
yathā bhavet suṣumṇāgā tathā bhavati khecarī // 146 //

Tr. Insert the tongue in the circle of *śṛṅkhalā.* As the tongue is able to enter *suṣumnā, khecarī* is perfected. 146.

Note: *Khecarī mudrā* has been greatly eulogized in *haṭhayogic* texts. There are six processes involved in the perfection of *khecarī mudrā* which are *chedana, cālana, dohana, manthana, praveśana* and *mantra.* The processes of *chedana, cālana* and *dohana* are to start simultaneously. *Manthana* or *gharṣaṇa* consists of rubbing with thumb on the four places, three times a day. The four places are frenum under the tongue, root of the tongue, palate and uvula. A detailed description of *khecarī* is found in MYS by *Ādinātha.*

These six verses (ii.141-146) seem to have been taken from *Khecarīpaṭala* as stated in AR (xxvii.4742-4745). 146.

खेचर्या मुद्रणे जाते देही देहं न मुञ्चति ॥
कायं[6] त्यक्त्वा तु कल्पान्ते ब्रह्मस्थानं व्रजत्यसौ ॥ 147 ॥

1. निर्मितां बरां–T,t1. 2. लम्बिकोत्पातकारिणीं –t1. 3. अनुपलब्धश्लोकः-P. 4. एतदनन्तरं – कपालकुहरे यस्तु ततो जिह्वां प्रवेशयेत् - अधिकः पाठः -P,T,t1. 5. भवेत्सुषुम्णागौ-P,T,t1. 6. कामं–P,T,t1.

khecaryā mudraṇe jāte dehī dehaṃ na muñcati //
kāyaṃ tyaktvā tu kalpānte brahmasthānaṃ vrajatyasau/147/

Tr. As the *khecarī* is attained, a mortal does not face (premature) death. Rather, at the end of a *kalpa*, he renounces the body and goes to *brahmasthāna.* 147.

प्राणे सुषुम्णा[1]सम्प्राप्ते नादं तु[2] श्रूयतेऽष्टधा ॥
घण्टादुन्दुभिशंखादि[3]वीणावेणुनिनादवत्[4] ॥
तनूनपात्तडित्तारेशपवनोपमम्[5] ॥ 148 ॥
prāṇe suṣumṇāsamprāpte nādaṃ tu śrūyate'ṣṭadhā //
ghaṇṭādundubhiśaṅkhādivīṇāveṇuninādavat //
tanūnapāttaḍittāreśapavanopamam // 148 //

Tr. When *prāṇa* enters into *suṣumnā*, eight types of *nādas* are heard, like sounds resembling that of a bell, trumpet, conch, *vīṇā,* flute, tiny bell, tinkling of a very fine pot, cracking sound of the fire, loud thunders and shrill sound of blowing air. 148.

वासुक्याद्यैश्च नागैश्च तक्षकेनाथवा पुनः ॥
दष्टस्य योगिनो देहे न विषं कर्तुमर्हति ॥ 149 ॥
vāsukyādyaiśca nāgaiśca takṣakenāthavā punaḥ //
daṣṭasya yogino dehe na viṣaṃ kartumarhati // 149 //

Tr. Such a *yogī,* even being bitten by (deadliest of) the serpents like *vāsukī, nāga* or *takṣaka,* will not be affected by poison. 149.

उत्कल्लोल[6]कलामृतं[7] च विमलं धारामृतं यः पिबेत् ॥
निर्दोषः स मृणालकोमलतनु[8]र्योगी चिरं जीवति ॥ 150 ॥
utkallolakalāmṛtaṃ ca vimalaṃ dhārāmṛtaṃ yaḥ pibet //
nirdoṣaḥ sa mṛṇālakomalatanuryogī ciraṃ jīvati // 150 //

---

1. सुषुम्नां–P,T,t1,n1,n3. 2.नादस्तु–P,T,n3. 3 . .शंखाभिः-P,T,t1,...शंखार्द्दे-N,J.
4 .वीणावेण्वग्नितालवत्-P,T,t1. 5. तनूनपात्रविस्तारतारेशपवनोपमम् -J,T,t1,n1,n2,n3,n4.
6 . तत्कल्लोल–N,n1,n4,J; उत्कंलोक-T. 7. कलभृतं–P. 8. वपुर्-P,T,t1.

Tr. The *yogī,* who sucks the divine ambrosia secreting from the moon, maintains the body as tender as the lotus stalk and lives long without diseases. 150.

सेवन्ते यदि लम्बिकाग्रमनिशं जिह्वा रसस्यन्दिनी
सक्षाराकटुतिक्तदुग्धसदृशं मध्वाज्यतुल्यं यदा[1] ‖ 151 ‖
sevante yadi lambikāgramaniśaṃ jihvā rasasyandinī //
sakṣārākaṭutiktadugdhasadṛśaṃ madhvājyatulyaṃ yadā /151/

Tr. The tip of the elongated tongue tastes the nectar, as salt, pungent, sour or milk, honey or ghee. 151.

अशेषाणां च नाडीनां जिह्वाग्रे रन्ध्रमागतः[2] ‖
विधत्ते[3] येन मार्गेण तेन चान्द्री[4] कलां व्रजेत् ‖ 152 ‖
aśeṣāṇāṃ ca nāḍīnāṃ jihvāgre randhramāgataḥ //
vidhatte yena mārgeṇa tena cāndrī kalāṃ vrajet // 152 //

Tr. Entire set of the *nāḍīs* has its base at the tip of the tongue, wherefrom the *yogī* enjoys (ambrosia oozing from *candra*). 152.

कन्यावादाखिला[5]वादरसवादादि[6]सिद्धयः ‖
योगिनः[7] सम्प्रवर्तन्ते तेषां वज्रोलि[8]खेचरी ‖ 153 ‖
kanyāvādākhilāvādarasavādādisiddhayaḥ //

yoginaḥ sampravartante teṣāṃ vajrolikhecarī // 153 //

Tr. All the *siddhis* attained through *kanyāvāda* (*kuṇḍalī*), *rasavāda* (alchemy) etc. are for those *yogīs* who attain *vajrolī* and *khecarī*. 153.

त्रिकटुम्बी[9] हठा चैव[10] गोलीढं[11] शिखरं तथा ‖
त्रिशंखी[12] वज्रमोंकारी[13] मूर्ध्वनालं[14] भुवोर्मुखे ‖ 154 ‖

---

1. मध्वाज्यतुल्याथवा–P,T,t1. 2. रन्ध्रगामता-N,n1,n3,n4,J,T,t1. 3. विद्यते-P,t1; विद्यन्ते-T. 4. चान्द्रीं–J, चाण्डीं -n1,n3. 5. बिलवाद–T,t1,n2. 6. रसवादस्तु–P,T. 7. योगिनां–P,T,t1. 8. वज्रोलि-J, वज्रली–T. 9. त्रिकुंड-P,T,t1. 10. सुचिहठा चैव-P,T,t1. 11. गोवीठं-P. 12. त्रिशंखि – P, श्रीशंखी –T,t1. 13. वज्रिमोंकारी-P,T,t1. 14. मूर्ध्वानालं-P,T,t1.

trikaṭumbī haṭhā caiva golīḍhaṃ śikharaṃ tathā //
triśaṅkhī vajramoṅkārī mūrdhvanālaṃ bhruvormukhe //154 //

Tr. The opening between two eyebrows is called *trikaṭumbī, haṭhā, golīḍha, śikhara, triśaṅkhī, vajra, oṃkārī, mūrdhvanāla*. 154.

पिंगला दम्भिनी[1] सूर्या यमिना काक्षरा[2] तथा[3] ॥
कालाग्निः रुद्री[4] चण्डी च[5] ते[6] स्युः पिंगलनामकाः[7] ॥ 155 ॥
piṅgalā dambhinī sūryā yaminā kākṣarā tathā //
kālāgniḥ rudrī caṇḍī ca te syuḥ piṅgalanāmakāḥ // 155 //

Tr. The synonyms of *piṅgalā* are: *piṅgalā, dambhinī, sūryā, yaminā, kākṣarā, kālāgni, rudrī* and *caṇḍī*. 155.

इडा चन्द्रा सिनीवाली[8] गंगा[9] चामरबोधिता[10] ॥
इडायाः वाचकाः शब्दाः पर्यायेण प्रकीर्तिताः ॥ 156 ॥
iḍā candrā sinīvālī gaṅgā cāmarabodhitā //
iḍāyāḥ vācakāḥ śabdāḥ paryāyeṇa prakīrtitāḥ // 156 //

Tr. The synonyms of *iḍā* are: *iḍā, candrā, sinīvālī, gaṅgā* and *amarabodhitā*. 156.

गोशब्देनोदिता जिह्वा तत्प्रवेशो हि[11] तालुनि ॥
गोमांसभक्षणं तत्तु महापातकनाशनम् ॥ 157 ॥
gośabdenoditā jihvā tatpraveśo hi tāluni //
gomāṃsabhakṣaṇaṃ tattu mahāpātakanāśanam // 157 //

Tr. The term '*go*' denotes tongue, which is to be inserted in the '*tālu*' (roof of the nasopharyngeal cavity). This literally means 'consuming *gomāṃsa*', which eliminates the severest of the sins. 157.

---

1. दुंभिनी-P. 2. यमिनाक्षरा-P; यमिकाक्षरा-T. 3. यथा –N,J. 4. कालाग्निरुद्री –P. 5. कालाग्नी रुद्रचण्डी च –T. 6. चेते -N,J. 7. पिंगलना तथा –T, अनुपलब्धपंक्तिः-t1. 8. चन्द्राशचीवाली -T; चन्द्राशशीवाली –P,t1. 9. गलगा –T,t1. 10. मधुबोधिता –T,t1; वामस्तुबोधिता -P. 11. अपि -P,T,t1.

गोमांसं भक्षयेन्नित्यं पिबेदमरवारुणीम् ॥
कुलीनं तमहं मन्ये अन्ये तु[1] कुलघातकाः ॥ 158 ॥
gomāṃsaṃ bhakṣayennityaṃ pibedamaravāruṇīm //
kulīnaṃ tamahaṃ manye anye tu kulaghātakāḥ // 158 //

Tr. I consider him the noble, who consumes '*gomāṃsa*' (insertion of the tongue) and sucks the divine ambrosia (secretion from the moon). Others are black-sheep. 158.

जिह्वाप्रवेशसम्भूत[2]वह्निनोत्थापिता[3] खलु ॥
चन्द्रात् स्रवति[4] यः सारः सा स्यादमरवारुणी ॥ 159 ॥[5]
jihvāpraveśasaṃbhūtavahninotthāpitā khalu //
candrāt sravati yaḥ sāraḥ sā syādamaravāruṇī //159 //

Tr. *Amara-vāruṇī* (the divine ambrosia) is the secretion of the nectar, which is made to flow from the moon by the stimulation of fire through insertion of the tongue in the cavity. 159.

इति श्रीनिवासयोगी[6]विरचितायां[7] हठरत्नावल्यां द्वितीयोपदेशः[8]

iti śrīnivāsayogīviracitāyāṃ haṭharatnāvalyāṃ dvitīyopadeśaḥ
This is the second chapter of Haṭharatnāvalī composed by Śrīnivāsayogī

---

1. इतरे P; त्वितरे –T,t1. 2. जिह्वाप्रवेशनं भूतं-P,T,t1. 3. वह्निनोद्दापिताखलु-P,T,t1, वह्निनोत्थापितः-n3. 4. द्रवति–T. 5. 'इति खेचरी मुद्रा'-P,T,t1. 6. योगीन्द्र-P,T. 7. श्रीनिवासविरचितायां–n2,n3,n4. 8. एतदनन्तरम्–
"वज्रोली वर—– दश महामुद्रान्वितैः कुम्भकैः
युक्तिः केवलकुम्भकेण महता क्षेमंकरेणाधिकम् ॥
ख्याते रम्यसुवर्णराजकथिते रत्नावलीनामके
ग्रन्थेऽस्मिन्नुपदेश एष विहितारम्भो (विविधारम्भो-t1) द्वितीयो गतः ॥"
अधिकः पाठः -P,T,t1.

हठरत्नावली

तृतीयोपदेशः[1]

अथाष्टांगयोगः[2]—
अथातोऽष्टांगयोगानां स्वरूपं किञ्चिदुच्यते[3] ॥
बहवो योगिनः सिद्धा अङ्गैरेतैश्च शोभनैः ॥ 1 ॥

athāṣṭāṅgayogaḥ —
athāto'ṣṭāṅgayogānāṃ svarūpaṃ kiñciducyate //
bahavo yoginaḥ siddhā aṅgairetaiśca śobhanaiḥ // 1 //

Tr. Now the nature of *aṣṭāṅga-yoga* is being explained. Many *yogīs* have attained *siddhis* through these efficacious methods. 1.

मनःप्रसादसन्तोषो मौनमिन्द्रियनिग्रहः ॥
दया दाक्षिण्यमास्तिक्यमार्जवं मार्द्दवं क्षमा ॥ 2 ॥
भावशुद्धिरहिंसा च ब्रह्मचर्यं स्मृतिर्धृतिः[4] ॥
इत्येवमादयश्चान्ये[5] मानसा[6] नियमाः स्मृताः ॥ 3 ॥

manaḥprasādasantoṣo maunamindriyanigrahaḥ //
dayā dākṣiṇyamāstikyamārjavaṃ mārddavaṃ kṣamā // 2 //
bhāvaśuddhirahiṃsā ca brahmacaryaṃ smṛtirdhṛtiḥ //
ityevamādayaścānye mānasā niyamāḥ smṛtāḥ // 3 //

Tr. Pacification of the mind, contentment, silence, control of sense organs, kindness, politeness, belief in God, straightforwardness, gentleness, forgiveness, purification of the thoughts, non-violence, celebacy, memory, forbearance and some such more—are known as *niyamas* for the mind. 2-3.

---

1. अनुपलब्धपाठः-N,J,P,T. 2. अष्टांगयोगमाह–J,n2, अथाष्टांगयोगमाह-P,J,T,n4, अनुपलब्धपाठः-P,T. 3. अनुपलब्धपाठः-N,n1,J, अनुपलब्धपंक्तिः-n2,n3,t1. 4. स्मृतिधृतिः-N. 5. इत्येवमाद्या येऽन्ये च–T,t1. 6. मनसो–P,T.

स्नानं शौचं ऋतं[1] सत्यं जप[2]होमश्च तर्पणम् ॥
तपोदान्तिस्तितिक्षा च नमस्कारः[3] प्रदक्षिणम् ॥
व्रतोपवासकाद्याश्च कायिका नियमाः स्मृताः ॥ 4 ॥

snānaṃ śaucaṃ vrataṃ satyaṃ japahomaśca tarpaṇam //
tapodāntistitikṣā ca namaskāraḥ pradakṣiṇam //
vratopavāsakādyāśca kāyikā niyamāḥ smṛtāḥ // 4 //

Tr. Bath, cleanliness, vow, truthfulness, recitation (of *mantras*), fire worship, libation of water, penance, self-control, endurance, reverential salutation, circumambulation, observance of vows, fasting etc.—are the *niyamas* for the body. 4.

Note: *Śrīnivāsa* introduces *aṣṭāṅgayoga*, but he has given only *niyamas* under two heads as *mānasa-niyama* and *kāyika-niyama*. He does not elaborate on *yamas* and *niyamas* separately. He has included *yamas* like *ahimsā* and *brahmacarya* in the *mānasa-niyamas*, while *satya* in *kāyika-niyamas*. The *niyamas* like *śauca*, *tapas* are included under *kāyika-niyamas*. This seems to be quite different type of classification under *niyamas*. 1-4.

हठस्य प्रथमांगत्वादासनं दर्श्यते[4] मया ॥
तत्कुर्यादासनं स्थैर्यमारोग्यं चांगपाटवम् ॥ 5 ॥
haṭhasya prathamāṅgatvādāsanaṃ darśyate mayā //
tatkuryādāsanaṃ sthairyamārogyaṃ cāṅgapāṭavam // 5 //

Tr. *Āsana*, being the first part of *haṭha-yoga* curriculam, is being narrated here by me. Practice of *āsanas* alleviates diseases and contributes to stability, health and efficient body.5.

वसिष्ठाद्यैश्च मुनिभि[5]र्मत्स्येन्द्राद्यैश्च योगिभिः ॥
अंगीकृतान्यासनानि लक्ष्यन्ते कानिचिन्मया[6] ॥ 6 ॥

---

1. व्रतं–J,N,n1,n3, शौचावृतं–T,t1. 2. जपो–t1. 3. नमस्कार–P,T,t1,n2. 4. लक्ष्यते-P,T,t1; दृश्यते–N,n1. 5. ' मुनिभिः'-अनुपलब्धपाठः-N,J. 6. अनुपलब्धपंक्तिः-n2,n4.

vasiṣṭhādyaiśca munibhirmatsyendrādyaiśca yogibhiḥ //
aṅgīkṛtānyāsanāni lakṣyante kānicinmayā // 6 //

Tr. Some of the *āsanas* accepted by the sages like *Vaśiṣṭha* and *yogīs* like *Matsyendra* are being described by me. 6.

Note: This verse is a repetition from HP and suggests two traditions of *āsanas*, namely, one of *munis* like *Vaśiṣṭha* etc., and the other of *yogīs* like *Matsyendra* etc. 6.

चतुरशीतिलक्षेषु एकैकं जीवजन्तुषु ॥
उद्धृत्य शम्भुना प्रोक्ताश्[1]चतुरशीति पीठिकाः[2] ॥ 7 ॥
caturaśītilakṣeṣu ekaikaṃ jīvajantuṣu //
uddhṛtya śambhunā proktāścaturaśīti pīṭhikāḥ // 7 //

Tr. *Śambhu* has culled only eighty four *āsanas* representing one from each lac of the eighty four lacs of species.7.

Note: It is customary in the *haṭha* texts, while describing *āsanas* to talk about the number of *āsanas* being eighty four lacs representing different species of creatures. GŚ (6) states that *Śiva* has enumerated eighty four *āsanas* representing one from each lac of the species. However, very few texts give the list of eighty four *āsanas*. This is one of the texts which enumerates eighty four *āsanas*. 7.

[3]चतुरशीतिपीठेषु[4] केषाञ्चिल्लक्षणं ब्रुवे ॥
आदिनाथोदिताः पीठाः देहारोग्यसुखप्रदाः ॥ 8 ॥
caturaśītipīṭheṣu keṣāñcillakṣaṇaṃ bruve //
ādināthoditāḥ pīṭhāḥ dehārogyasukhapradāḥ // 8 //

Tr. From among eighty four *pīṭhas*, I give the characteristics of a few. These *pīṭhas* are recommended by *Ādinātha*, and contribute to the sense of wellbeing. 8.

Note: *Śrīnivāsa* has used *pīṭha* as a synonym for *āsana*. Although *Śrīnivāsa* enumerates eighty four *āsanas* in further verses, he does not describe the techniques of all the *āsanas*.

---

1. ' मत्स्येन्द्राद्यैश्च —शम्भुना प्रोक्ताश्' –अनुपलब्धः –J,N,n1,n2,n3. 2. पीठकाः-J,P, चतुरशीतपीठिका–n2. 3. चतुरशीतिपीठकाः-t1,n4. 4. पीठानां–P,T,t1.

JP also describes eighty four *āsanas*, but most of the names vary from the list given by *Śrīnivāsa*. 8.

सिद्धं भद्रं[1] तथा[2] वज्रं सिंह[3]शिल्पासनं परम् ॥[4]
बन्धं करः[5] सम्पुटितं[6] शुद्धं[7] पद्मचतुष्टयम्[8] ॥ 9 ॥
दण्डपार्श्वं[9] च सहजं बन्धपिण्डं मयूरकम् ॥
एकपादं मयूरं[10] च षण्मयूरमिहोच्यते ॥ 10 ॥
भैरवं कामदहनं पाणिपात्रं च कार्मुकम् ॥
स्वस्तिकं गोमुखं वीरं मण्डूकं[11] मर्कटासनम् ॥ 11 ॥
मत्स्येन्द्रं पार्श्वमत्स्येन्द्रं बद्ध[12]मत्स्येन्द्रमेव च ॥
निरालम्बनं[13] चान्द्राख्यं[14] काण्ठवं[15] चैकपादकम् ॥ 12 ॥
फणीन्द्रं पश्चिमं तानं[16] शयितपश्चिमतानकम्[17] ॥
करणी चित्रनामासौ योगनिद्रा[18] विधूननम्[19] ॥ 13 ॥[20]
पादपीडन[21]हंसाख्ये[22] नाभीतलमतःपरम् ॥
आकाशमुत्पादतलं नाभीलसितपादकम् ॥ 14 ॥[20]
वृश्चिकासनं चक्राख्य[23]मुत्फालकमितीर्यते ॥
उत्तानकूर्मं कूर्मं च बद्धकूर्मं च नार्जवम्[24] ॥ 15 ॥
कबन्धासनमित्याहुः गोरक्षासनमेव च ॥
अंगुष्ठमुष्टिकं ज्ञेयं[25] ब्रह्मप्रासादितं[26] तथा ॥ 16 ॥
पञ्चचूलिं[27] कुक्कुटं च एकपादककुक्कुटम् ॥
आकारितं बन्धचूली पार्श्वकुक्कुटमेव च ॥ 17 ॥

---

1. पद्मं–n2,n3,n4. 2. करं–T. 3. सिंहं-n2,n3,n4. 4. सिद्धं भ्रदं वज्रसिंह शिल्पसिहासनं परम्'-P,T,t1. 5. बन्धकरं–n2, करं–t1. 6. बन्धं करसम्पुटितं–P,T,J,n1,n3,n4. 7. बन्धकरसम्पुटितशुद्धपद्मं–P, शुद्धपद्मं–T,t1. 8. शुद्धपद्मचतुष्टयं–n2. 9. दत्तपार्श्व -J,N,n3; दन्तपार्श्व-T,n1. 10. एकपादमयूरं–P,T,t1,n2. 11. माण्डूकं–P,T. 12. बन्ध–P,T,t1. 13. निरालम्बन–P,t1. 14. सान्द्राक्षौ–N,n1,n2,n3,J; शाद्राख्यं-T,t1, निरालम्बनसान्द्राक्षौ–n4. 15. भौण्डवं–N,n1,n3,n4,J. 16. ताणेः-t1. 17. शैतपश्चिमतानकम्-T,t1. 18. योगमुद्रा–P,T,N,J. 19. वधानने-T,t1. 20. श्लोक संख्या 12 तथा 13 अनुपलब्धा-N,n1,n2,n3,n4,J. 21. पादपिण्डन–t1. 22. पादपिण्डनहिंसाख्ये–P,T. 23. वृश्चिकासनचक्राख्ये –P,T,t1. 24 वनार्जवम्-J. 25. अंगुष्ठमुष्ठिकाज्ञेये–T,t1. 26. ब्रह्मप्रासारितं-N,J,t1. 27. पञ्चूचूली–J,N,n2,n3,n4,t1, पञ्चचूली–P,T.

अर्धनारीश्वरश्चैते[1] बकासन[2]धरावहे ॥
चन्द्रकान्तं[3] सुधासारं[4] व्याघ्रासनमतः[5] परम् ॥ 18 ॥
राजासनमथेन्द्राणी शरभासनमेव च ॥
रत्नासनं चित्रपीठं बद्धपक्षीश्वरासनम् ॥ 19 ॥
विचित्र[6]नलिनं कान्तं शुद्धपक्षी सुमन्द्रकम्[7] ॥
चौरंगी च[8] तथा[9] क्रौञ्चं दृढासनखगासने ॥
ब्रह्मासनं नागपीठमन्तिमं च शवासनम्[10] ॥ 20 ॥
एवं मिलित्वा चतुरशीत्यासनानि[11] ॥

siddhaṃ bhadraṃ tathā vajraṃ siṃhaśilpāsanaṃ param //
bandhaṃ karaḥ samputitaṃ śuddhaṃ padmacatuṣṭayam / 9 /
daṇḍapārśvaṃ ca sahajaṃ bandhapiṇḍaṃ mayūrakam //
ekapādaṃ mayūraṃ ca ṣaṇmayūramihocyate //10 //
bhairavaṃ kāmadahanaṃ pāṇipātraṃ ca kārmukam //
svastikaṃ gomukhaṃ vīraṃ maṇḍūkaṃ markaṭāsanam /11//
matsyendrampārśvamatsyendraṃ baddhamatsyendrameva ca
nirālambanaṃ cāndrākhyaṃ kāṇṭhavaṃ caikapādakam //12 //
phaṇīndraṃ paścimaṃ tānaṃ śayitapaścimatānakam //
karaṇī citranāmāsau yoganidrā vidhūnanam // 13 //
pādapīḍanaṃ haṃsākhye nābhītalamataḥparam //
ākāśamutpādatalaṃ nābhīlasitapādakam // 14 //
vṛścikāsanaṃ cakrākhyamutphālakamitīryate //
uttānakūrmaṃ kūrmaṃ ca baddhakūrmaṃ ca nārjavam /15 //
kabandhāsanamityāhuḥ gorakṣāsanameva ca //
aṅguṣṭhamuṣṭikaṃ jñeyaṃ brahmaprāsāditaṃ tathā // 16 //
pañcacūliṃ kukkuṭaṃca ekapādakakukkuṭam //
ākāritaṃ bandhacūlī pārśvakukkuṭameva ca // 17 //
ardhanārīśvaraścaite bakāsanadharāvahe //
candrakāntaṃ sudhāsāraṃ vyāghrāsanamataḥ param // 18 //

---

1. अर्द्ध-नारीश्वर ' चैते–P,T,t1. 2. वकासनं–T1J,n1,n2,n3,n4. 3. चन्द्रकान्त-P.
4. सुरासारं –N,n3,J. 5. मितः -P,T,t1. 6. विचित्रं –P. 7. सुमन्दकम् -P,T,t1,n1,n2,n3.
8. चौरण्डकं –n3. 9. चौरं —तथा –J,n1, चौरासनं तथा –N. 10. शरासनं –T,t1.
11. अनुपलब्धपंक्तिः-J,N,n1,n2,n3.

tatra siddhāsanam—
yonisthānakamaṅghrimūlaghaṭitaṃ kṛtvā dṛḍhaṃ vinyasen
meḍhre pādamathaikameva niyataṃ kṛtvā samaṃ vigraham //
sthāṇuḥ saṃyamitendriyo'caladṛśā paśyan bhruvorantaraṃ
caitanmokṣakapāṭabhedajanakaṃ śiddhāsanaṃ procyate / 25/

Tr. One should press the heel firmly against the perineum and place the other foot over the genital. He should remain straight and steady, control the senses, and keep the gaze fixed between the eyebrows. This is *siddhāsana,* which opens the door to liberation (*mokṣa*). 25.

मतान्तरे तु[1] —
मेढ्रादुपरि निःक्षिप्य[2] सव्यं गुल्फं[3] तथोपरि ॥
गुल्फान्तरं तु[4] निःक्षिप्य सिद्धाः सिद्धासनं विदुः ॥ 26 ॥

matāntare tu —
meḍhrādupari niḥkṣipya savyaṃ gulphaṃ tathopari //
gulphāntaraṃ tu niḥkṣipya siddhāḥ siddhāsanaṃ viduḥ //26 //

According to others—

Tr. One places the left ankle over the genital and the other ankle over the first one. According to the *siddhas*, this is *siddhāsana*. 26.

एतत्सिद्धासनं प्राहुरन्ये वज्रासनं विदुः ॥
मुक्तासनं वदन्त्यन्ये[5] प्राहुर्गुप्तासनं परे ॥ 27 ॥
etat siddhāsanaṃ prāhuranye vajrāsanaṃ viduḥ //
muktāsanaṃ vadantyanye prāhurguptāsanaṃ pare // 27 //

Tr. This same *siddhāsana* is variously known as *vajrāsana, muktāsana* and *guptāsana* by others. 27.

Note: Although in this verse, *vajrāsana, muktāsana* and *guptāsana* are considered synonyms of *siddhāsana*, other authorities, however, make differentiation in these four variations of *siddhāsana.*

---

1. अनुपलब्धपाठः-N,n1,2,3,J. 2. विन्यस्य-P,T,t1. 3. सव्यगुल्फं–n2. 4. च-P,T,t1.
5. वदन्त्येके-P,T,t1,n2.

1. When left heel is placed at the perineum and the right heel is placed on the organ of generation, it is *siddhāsana*.
2. When right heel is placed at the perineum and the left heel is placed on the organ of generation, it is *vajrāsana*.
3. When the right heel is placed on the left heel and both the heels are placed at the perineum, it is *muktāsana*.
4. When right heel is placed on the left heel and both the heels are placed on the organ of generation, it is *guptāsana*.

GhS (ii.20) gives another technique of *guptāsana*, in which one hides the two feet between the knees and thighs in such a manner that the feet come under the anus. 27.

ब्रह्मचारी मिताहारी त्यागी[1] योगपरायणः ॥
अब्दादूर्ध्वं भवेत्सिद्धो[2] नात्र कार्या विचारणा ॥ 28 ॥

brahmacārī mitāhārī tyāgī yogaparāyaṇaḥ //
abdādūrdhvaṃ bhavetsiddho nātra kāryā vicāraṇā // 28 //

Tr. There is no doubt that one, who observes celibacy, consumes moderate food, is detached (to worldy objects) and devoted to *yoga*, attains success after one year. 28.

नासनं सिद्धसदृशं न कुम्भकं केवलोपमः[3] ॥
न खेचरीसमा[4] मुद्रा न नादसदृशो लयः ॥ 29 ॥

nāsanaṃ siddhasadṛśaṃ na kumbhakaṃ kevalopamaḥ //
na khecarīsamā mudrā na nādasadṛśo layaḥ // 29 //

Tr. There is no *āsana* like *siddha*, no *kumbhaka* like *kevala*, no *mudrā* like *khecarī* and no *laya* (absorption) like *nāda*. 29.

---

1. योगी-P,T,t1. 2. भवेत्सिद्धिः-P,T,t1. 3. नासनं सिद्धसदृशं न कुंभसदृशोऽनिलः-N,n1,n2,n3,J. 4. खेचर्या समा –P,T,t1.

अथ भद्रासनम् —
गुल्फौ च वृषणस्याधः सीवन्याः[1] पार्श्वयाः क्षिपेत् ॥
पार्श्वपादौ[2] च पाणिभ्यां दृढं बद्ध्वा सुनिश्चलम्[3] ॥
भद्रासनं भवेदेतत् सर्वव्याधिविषापहम् ॥ 30 ॥

atha bhadrāsanam —
gulphau ca vṛṣaṇasyādhaḥ sīvanyāḥ pārśvayoḥ kṣipet //
pārśvapādau ca pāṇibhyāṃ dṛḍhaṃ baddhvā suniścalam //
bhadrāsanaṃ bhavedetat sarvavyādhiviṣāpaham // 30 //

Tr. The two ankles are put under the scrotum on the two sides of the perineum. One catches hold of the feet with hands and remains steady. This is *bhadrāsana,* which removes all the diseases and toxins. 30.

Note: GhS(ii.9-10) gives a different variety of *bhadrāsana*. In this, instead of two ankles placed on the two respective sides of the perineum, the ankles are everted with the toes turned backwards. For detailed discussion, refer to YM (vol. x, No. 1, pp.28-33). 30.

अथ सिंहासनम्[4] —
गुल्फौ च वृषणस्याधः सीवन्याः[5] पार्श्वयोः क्षिपेत् ॥ [4]
दक्षिणे सव्यगुल्फं च दक्षिणे तु तथेतरम्[6] ॥ 31 ॥
हस्तौ च जान्वोः[7] संस्थाप्य स्वाङ्गुलीः[8] सम्प्रसार्य च ॥
व्यात्तवक्त्रो निरीक्षेत नासाग्रं सुसमाहितः ॥ 32 ॥

atha siṃhāsanam–
gulphau ca vṛṣaṇasyādhaḥ sīvanyāḥ pārśvayoḥ kṣipet //
dakṣiṇe savyagulphaṃ ca dakṣiṇe tu tathetaram // 31 //
hastau ca jānvoḥ saṃsthāpya svāṅgulīḥ samprasārya ca //
vyāttavaktro nirīkṣeta nāsāgraṃ susamāhitaḥ // 32 //

---

1. स्विवन्यां –T. 2. पार्श्वे पादौ-P,T,t1. 3. सुनिश्चलां –P,t1. 4. अनुपलब्धपंक्तिः-T. 5. सीवन्यां –P, स्विवन्यां –t1. 6. दक्षिणे सव्यगुल्फं तु दक्षगुल्फं तु वामके -P,T,t1,n2. 7. जानौ-N,J. 8. स्वाङ्गुलीं-P,T,t1.

Tr. The ankles are placed under the scrotum on both the sides of the perineum in such a manner that the left ankle is on the right side and the right on the left. The palms are placed on the knees, spreading the fingers and the mouth kept wide open. One fixes the gaze on the tip of the nose. 31-32.

सिंहासनं भवेदेतत्सेवितं[1] योगिभिः सदा ॥
बन्धत्रितयसंस्थानं कुरुते चासनोत्तमम् ॥ 33 ॥

siṃhāsanaṃ bhavedetatsevitaṃ yogibhiḥ sadā //
bandhatritayasaṃsthānaṃ kurute cāsanottamam // 33 //

Tr. This is *siṃhāsana* practised by all the *yogīs*. This is an excellent *āsana*, which facilitates the application of the three *bandhas*. 33.

अथ पद्मासनम् —
वामोरूपरि दक्षिणं च चरणं संस्थाप्य वामं तथा
याम्योरूपरि पश्चिमेन विधिना धृत्वा कराभ्यां दृढम् ॥
अंगुष्ठौ[2] हृदये निधाय चिबुकं[3] नासाग्रमालोकयेद्
एतद् व्याधिविनाशकारि[4] यमिनां[5] पद्मासनं प्रोच्यते ॥ 34 ॥

***atha padmāsanam* —**
vāmorūpari dakṣiṇaṃ ca caraṇaṃ saṃsthāpya vāmaṃ tathā
yāmyorūpari paścimena vidhinā dhṛtvā karābhyāṃ dṛḍham //
aṅguṣṭhau hṛdaye nidhāya cibukaṃ nāsāgramālokayed
etad vyādhivināśakāri yamināṃ padmāsanaṃ procyate /34/

Tr. The right foot is placed on the left thigh and the left on the right, the big toes are held with the respective hands crossed behind the back, chin pressed against the chest and the gaze is directed towards the tip of the nose. This is *padmāsana*, which alleviates diseases of the *yogīs*. 34.

---

1. भवेदेतत् भजन्तं-P,T,t1, सेविते–T,n3,n4. 2. अंगुष्ठं-P,T,t1. 3. चुबुकं–T,t1.
4. एतद्व्याधिविनाशी–t1. 5. नाशनकरं–n3.

Note: The *padmāsana* described here and also in GhS (ii.8) and GŚ (9) is popularly known as *baddhapadmāsana*. TBU (*mantra*- 39-40) describes *padmāsana* and *baddhapadmāsana* separately. 34.

तथा च याज्ञवल्क्यः —

पादाङ्गुष्ठौ[1] निबध्नीया[2]द्धस्ताभ्यां व्युत्क्रमेण[3] तु ॥
ऊर्वोरुपरि विप्रेन्द्र कृत्वा पादतले उभे ॥
पद्मासनं भवेदेतत् सर्वेषामपि पूजितम्[4] ॥ 35 ॥

***tathā ca yājñavalkyaḥ* —**

pādāṅguṣṭhau nibadhnīyāddhastābhyāṃ vyutkrameṇa tu //
ūrvorupari viprendra kṛtvā pādatale ubhe //
padmāsanaṃ bhavedetat sarveṣāmapi pūjitam // 35 //

According to *Yājñavalkya* —

Tr. Place both the feet on the opposite thighs and catch hold of the big toes with the respective hands crossed. This is *padmāsana* respected by all. 35.

दत्तात्रेयोऽपि —

उत्तानौ चरणौ[5] कृत्वा ऊर्वोः संस्थाप्य यत्नतः ॥
ऊरुमध्ये तथोत्तानौ[6] पाणी[7] कृत्वा ततो दृशौ ॥ 36 ॥
नासाग्रे विन्यसेद्राजदन्तमूलं च[8] जिह्वया ॥
उत्तम्भ्य चिबुकं[9] वक्षःसंस्थाप्य पवनं शनैः ॥ 37 ॥

***dattātreyo'pi* —**

uttānau caraṇau kṛtvā ūrvoḥ saṃsthāpya yatnataḥ //
ūrumadhye tathottānau pāṇī kṛtvā tato dṛśau // 36 //
nāsāgre vinyasedrājadantamūlaṃ ca jihvayā //
uttambhya cibukaṃ vakṣaḥsaṃsthāpya
pavanaṃ śanaiḥ //37//

---

1. पादांगुष्ठौ च-P, पदांगुष्ठौ न–t1. 2. निबध्नीया-T; बध्नीया-P,t1. 3. क्रमेण-P,T,t1. 4. पूज्यते -P,T. 5. चरणौ –अनुपलब्धः –N. 6. ततो स्थानौ -P; ततोत्थानौ-T. 7. पाणिं –J,N. 8. तु-P,T,t1,n2. 9. चुबुके –P,T,t1.

According to *Dattātreya*—

Tr. Firmly place the upturned feet on the opposite thighs. Place the upturned palms between the thighs. Fix the gaze on the tip of the nose. Press the tongue against the root of the front teeth, press the chin against the chest and gently raise the *pavana* (*prāṇa*) up. 36-37.

इदं पद्मासनं प्रोक्तं सर्वव्याधिविनाशनम्[1] ॥
दुर्लभं येन केनापि धीमता लभ्यते भुवि ॥ 38 ॥
idaṃ padmāsanaṃ proktaṃ sarvavyādhivināśanam //
durlabhaṃ yena kenāpi dhīmatā labhyate bhuvi // 38 //

Tr. This is *padmāsana*, which cures all the diseases. This is difficult to be attained even by the wise. 38.

Note: In the earlier verse, there is a specific mention of placing the right foot on the left thigh and the left foot on the right thigh. Here there is no such mention. It only suggests that the feet should be on the opposite thighs and hands are placed one over the other. In this technique *jālandhara bandha* is to be accompanied with *jihvābandha*. There is no mention of *uḍḍiyāna bandha*. *brahmānanda*, commenting on this verse in HP(i.47), suggests that *jālandhara bandha* accompanied with *jihvā bandha* alone serves the purpose of *mūlabandha* and *uḍḍiyāna bandha*. 36-38.

कृत्वा सम्पुटितौ करौ दृढतरं बद्ध्वा[2] तु पद्मासनम्
गाढं वक्षसि सन्निधाय[3] चिबुकं[4] ध्यानं च तच्चेतसि ॥
वारंवारमपानमूर्ध्वमनिलं प्रोच्चारयेत्[5] पूरितम्
मुञ्चत्प्राणमुपैति बोधमतुलं शक्तेः प्रभावान्नरः ॥ 39 ॥

kṛtvā samputitau karau dṛḍhataraṃ baddhvā tu padmāsanam
gāḍhaṃ vakṣasi sannidhāya cibukaṃ dhyānaṃ ca taccetasi //
vāraṃvāramapānamūrdhvamanilaṃ proccārayet pūritam
muñcatprāṇamupaiti bodhamatulaṃ śakteḥ prabhāvānnaraḥ // 39//

---

1. सर्वव्याधिनिवारणम् -P,T,t1. 2. कृत्वा –N,J. 3. संविधाय –J,n2. 4. चुबुके –N,J,t1. 5. प्रोच्चालयत् -P,T,t1,n2.

Tr. Firmly adopt *padmāsana*, fold the hands, firmly press the chin against the chest and repeatedly raise the *apāna* upwards forcefully so that it unites with *prāṇa*. Thus, one attains unparallel wisdom of the highest order through the arousal of *śakti (kuṇḍalī)* and by intense concentration on the Supreme Reality. 39.

Note: This verse is included under the description of *mudrās* in HP (10 ch. v. 145) published by Lonavla Yoga Institute (India). 39.

पद्मासने स्थितो[1] योगी नाडीद्वारेषु पूरयेत् ॥
पूरितं ध्रियते यस्तु[2] स मुक्तो[3] नात्र संशयः ॥ 40 ॥
padmāsane sthito yogī nāḍīdvāreṣu pūrayet //
pūritaṃ dhrīyate yastu sa mukto nātra saṃśayaḥ // 40 //

Tr. Adopting *padmāsana*, a *yogī* should inhale through the two nostrils and hold the breath. Thus one undoubtedly becomes liberated. 40.

करौ सम्पुटितौ कुर्यात् तत्सम्पुटितपंकजम् ॥ 41 ॥
karau saṃpuṭitau kuryāt tat saṃpuṭitapaṅkajam // 41 //

Tr. When palms are folded forming a cavity, it is *saṃpuṭita-paṅkaja*. 41.

Note: *Śrīnivāsa*, while commenting on the *āsanas*, gives four types of *padmāsanas*, namely, *baddhapadmāsana, karapadma, saṃ puṭitapadma,* and *śuddhapadma*, but he does not describe all of them. 41.

अथ मयूरम्[4] –

धरामवष्टभ्य करद्वयेन तत्कूपरि[5] स्थापितनाभिपार्श्वः ॥
उच्चासनो दण्डवदुत्थितः खे मयूरमेतत्प्रवदन्ति[6] पीठम् ॥ 42 ॥

---

1. पद्मासनस्थितो –P,T,t1. 2. पूरितं क्रियते यस्तु -P; मारुतं पीयते येन -N. 3. भुक्तो –P. 4. मायूरम् -P,N,n1,n2,n3,T. 5. तत्कूर्पर -P, करस्थूलाभ्यां तत्कूर्पर –T,t1. 6. मायूरमेतत् -P,t1, मायूरमेतद्वदन्ति -T.

atha mayūram —

dharāmavaṣṭabhya karadvayena
tatkūrpare sthāpitanābhipārśvaḥ //
uccāsano daṇḍavadutthitaḥ khe
mayūrametat pravadanti pīṭham // 42 //

Tr. The two palms are placed on the ground. Elbows are placed on the respective sides of the navel and the body is lifted in the air like a horizontal stick. This is known as *mayūra-pīṭha*. 42.

हरति सकलरोगानाशु गुल्मोदरादीन्
अभिभवति च[1] दोषानासनं श्रीमयूरम् ॥
बहुकदशनभुक्तं भस्मकुर्याद्विचित्रम्
जनयति जठराग्निं जीर्यते कालकूटम् ॥ 43 ॥

harati sakalarogānāśu gulmodarādīn
abhibhavati ca doṣānāsanaṃ śrīmayūram //
bahukadaśanabhuktaṃ bhasmakuryādvicitraṃ
janayati jaṭharāgniṃ jīryate kālakūṭam // 43 //

Tr. *Mayūrāsana* enables quick relief from all the diseases of the spleen and the stomach and cures the imbalances caused by the humours. It further digests excess food and bad food, stimulates gastric fire and even digests the deadly poison. 43.

मयूरं दण्डवत्कुर्यान्मायूरं[2] दण्डनामकम्[3] ॥
कुर्यान्मायूरं पार्श्वाभ्यां मायूरपार्श्वनामकम्[4] ॥ 44 ॥

mayūraṃ daṇḍavatkuryānmāyūraṃ daṇḍanāmakam //
kuryānmāyūraṃ pārśvābhyāṃ māyūrapārśvanāmakam //44//

Tr. When *mayūra* is practised like a (horizontal) stick, it is called *daṇḍa-māyūra*. This same when practised on both the sides, is *pārśva-māyūra*. 44.

---

1. च- अनुपलब्धः–J,T. 2. मयूरं –T. 3. दण्डवन्मतम् -J,n3, दण्डवर्त्मकम्-n2. 4. मायूरं पार्श्व नामकम्-P, मायूरं पार्श्वनामवत् -T,t1.

मयूरं[1] पद्मकं कुर्यात् बद्धकेकीति[2] कथ्यते ॥ 45 ॥
mayūraṃ padmakaṃ kuryāt baddhakekīti kathyate // 45 //

Tr. With *padmāsana, mayūra* is called *baddhakekī*. 45.

अथ पिण्डमयूरासनम्[3] —
एकं पादं[4] मयूराग्रे प्रसार्यैकं मयूरवत्[5] ॥
इदं पिण्ड[6]मयूराख्यं सर्वव्याधिविनाशकम्[7] ॥ 46 ॥
atha piṇḍamayūrāsanam —
ekaṃ pādaṃ mayūrāgre prasāryaikaṃ mayūravat //
idaṃ piṇḍamayūrākhyaṃ sarvavyādhivināśakam // 46 //

Tr. Stretch one leg infront and the other stretched out like a peacock. This is *piṇḍa-mayūra,* which cures all the ailments. 46.

एकपादमयूरासनम्[8] —
कण्ठे पादं[9] प्रसार्यैकमेकपादं[10] मयूरके ॥ 47 ॥
ekapādamayūrāsanam —
kaṇṭhe pādaṃ prasāryaikamekapādaṃ mayūrake // 47 //

Tr. One leg is placed over the neck and the other stretched out, forming *ekapāda-mayūra*. 47.

Note: *Śrīnivāsa* gives six varieties of *mayūrāsana* but describes only five. The *sahajamayūra* has not been described. 47.

अथ भैरवासनम् —
गुल्फौ सम्पीड्य चान्योऽन्यं व्युत्क्रमेणोत्थितं शनैः ॥
जान्वोः पार्श्वगतौ हस्तौ दण्डवद् भैरवासनम् ॥ 48 ॥
atha bhairavāsanam —
gulphau sampīḍya cānyo'nyaṃ vyutkrameṇotthitaṃ śanaiḥ //
jānvoḥ pārśvagatau hastau daṇḍavad bhairavāsanam // 48 //

Tr. Press the two ankles with each other and raise them up. Place the hands straight by the sides of the knees. This is *bhairavāsana*. 48.

---

1. मायूरं–T,n3. 2. बंधेकेकीति-N,J, बद्धकेकेति-T. 3. पिण्डमयूरम्-P,T,J,n2. 4. एकपादं–N,P,T. 5. मयूरतः-P,T,t1. 6. पिण्डं–P. 7. विनाशनम्-P,T. 8. अनुपलब्धः–J,T,n1,n2,n3. 9. पदं-P. 10. प्रसार्यैकपादं-n1,n2,n3,n4,T1; प्रसायैव एकपादं-T.

अथ कामदहनम्[1] —
भद्रासनं सुखं स्थाप्य विपरीते तु द्वे पदे[2] ॥
अनेन यदि कुर्याच्चैतत्[3] कामदहनं[4] भवेत् ॥ 49 ॥
atha kāmadahanam —
bhadrāsanaṃ sukhaṃ sthāpya viparīte tu dve pade //
anena yadi kuryāccaitat kāmadahanaṃ bhavet // 49 //

Tr. Comfortably adopt *bhadrāsana* and place the toes turned backwards. This posture is *kāmadahana*. 49.

Note: The arrangement of the feet resembles the technique of *bhadrāsana* described in GhS (ii.9-10). 49.

अथ पाणिपात्रासनम्[5] —
नाभौ संस्थाप्य गुल्फौ च तन्मध्ये करपात्रताम् ॥
शनैर्यत्नेन कुर्वीत पाणिपात्रं तदुच्यते ॥ 50 ॥
atha pāṇipātrāsanam —
nābhau saṃsthāpya gulphau ca tanmadhye karapātratām //
śanairyatnena kurvīta pāṇipātraṃ taducyate // 50 //

Tr. Gently press the ankles against the navel and arrange the hands like a water pot there. This is *pāṇipātra*. 50.

अथ धनुरासनम् —
पादांगुष्ठौ तु पाणिभ्यां गृहीत्वा श्रवणावधि ॥
धनुराकर्षणं कृत्वा[6] धनुरासनमुच्यते[7] ॥ 51 ॥
atha dhanurāsanam —
pādāṅguṣṭhau tu pāṇibhyāṃ gṛhītvā śravaṇāvadhi //
dhanurākarṣaṇaṃ kṛtvā dhanurāsanamucyate // 51 //

Tr. The big toes are held with the hands and are pulled upto the ears (alternately). Thus, one assumes the shape of a stretched bow. This is *dhanurāsana*. 51.

---

1. अथ कामदहनासनम्-n1. 2. पदोः-J,P,T, पदौ–n2, पदयोः -n3. 3. कुर्याद्वि-P,t1, कुर्याद्वे-T. 4. तत्कामदहनो-N,J,t1. 5. पाणिपात्रे-J, पाणिपात्रम् -P,T,n2. 6. धनुशकर्षणाकृष्टं-P; धनुराकारणाकृष्टं-T,t1. 7. धनुरासनमेव च-P.

Note: This variety is called *ākarṣaṇa-dhanurāsana* to differentiate it from the variety of *dhanurāsana* described in GhS (ii.18). The technique of *dhanurāsana* described in GhS is different and is done in prone lying position. For detailed discussion, see YM (vol.ix, No. 4, pp. 42-54). 51.

अथ स्वस्तिकासनम् —
जानूर्वोरन्तरं सम्यक् कृत्वा पादतले उभे ॥
ऋजुकायसमासीनः[1] स्वस्तिकं तत्प्रचक्षते ॥ 52 ॥[2]

atha svastikāsanam —
jānūrvorantaraṃ samyak kṛtvā pādatale ubhe //
ṛjukāyasamāsīnaḥ svastikaṃ tat pracakṣate // 52 //

Tr. Arrange both the soles (feet) properly between the thighs and the shanks and sit erect. This is called *svastikāsana.* 52.

Note: *Brahmānanda* in his commentary *Jyotsnā* suggests the reading '*jaṅghorvor*' instead of '*jānūrvor*', meaning 'between the thigh and the shank', rather than 'thigh and the knee'. 52.

अथ गोमुखासनम् —
सव्ये दक्षिणगुल्फं तु पृष्ठपार्श्वे नियोजयेत् ॥
दक्षिणेऽपि तथा सव्यं गोमुखं गोमुखासनम्[3] ॥ 53 ॥

atha gomukhāsanam —
savye dakṣiṇagulphaṃ tu pṛṣṭhapārśve niyojayet //
dakṣiṇe'pi tathā savyaṃ gomukhaṃ gomukhāsanam // 53 //

Tr. Place the right ankle by the side of the left hip and the left ankle by the right hip, thus imitating the shape of a cow's head. This is *gomukhāsana.* 53.

Note: Another popular variety of *gomukhāsana* requires the hands to be braced on the back, left hand coming from below and the right hand coming from above over the right shoulder. This

---

1. ऋजुकायः सुखासीनः-P,T,t1, ऋजुकायः समासीनः-n3. 2. श्लोकोऽयं गोमुखासनानन्तरं-P. 3. गोमुखाकृति-P.

arrangement of the hands is described in BYS-19,20 and generally it is practised. This may be called *baddhahasta-gomukhāsana*. HY, however, suggests to hold the big toes by crossing the hands behind. For detailed discussion on varieties of *gomukhāsana*, refer to YM (vol.xviii, No. 1, pp.41-44). 53.

अथ वीरासनम्[1] —
एकं पादमथैकस्मिन् विन्यसेदूरुणि स्थिरम्[2] ॥
इतरस्मिंस्तथा चोरुं[3] **वीरासनमितीरितम्** ॥ 54 ॥[4]

atha vīrāsanam —
ekaṃ pādamathaikasmin vinyasedūruṇi sthiram //
itarasmiṃstathā coruṃ vīrāsanamitīritam // 54 //

Tr. Place one foot on the opposite thigh and the other foot above the opposite thigh and remain steady. This is called *vīrāsana*. 54.

Note: This is also known as *ardhāsana* in YV (II: 46). Besides HP(i.21), this variety is described in other *yogic* texts such as SUp (i: 2-4), TBU (37), AhS (xxxi: 39) and TVd (ii: 46). The technique of *vīrāsana* differs in GhS(ii.17) from the one given here. In GhS variety, one foot is placed on the opposite thigh while turning the other foot backwards. Traditions differ in the use of the upper foot being placed on the opposite thigh. JUp (iii: 6) prescribes left foot to be kept on the right thigh, while *Brahmānanda* in his commentary *Jyotsnā*, recommends right foot to be placed on the left thigh. But HP permits both these variations. Although, there is no mention about the arrangement of hands in *vīrāsana*, its being a meditative pose, the hands are comfortably placed on the knees. 54.

अथ मण्डूकासनम्[5] —
पृष्ठं[6] **सम्पीड्य गुल्फाभ्यां जान्वंगे सवलयाकृतिः**[7] ॥
हस्तौ पादतले क्षिप्तौ मण्डूकं पाददोषहृत् ॥ 55 ॥

---

1. अनुपलब्धः–J. 2. स्थितं–T. 3. इतरेऽस्मिन् तथा चोक्तं–T,t1. 4. अनुपलब्धः-N,n1,n2,n3,J. 5. अनुपलब्धः-N,n1,n2,n3,J. 6. पादौ-P. 7. सरलाकृतिः-N,n1,n3,J.

***atha maṇḍūkāsanam* —**
pṛṣṭhaṃ sampīḍya gulphābhyāṃ jānvaṅge savalayākṛtiḥ //
hastau pādatale kṣiptau maṇḍūkaṃ pādadoṣahṛt // 55 //

Tr. The ankles are placed under the buttocks. The knees are kept wide apart. Hands are placed under the feet. This is *maṇḍūkāsana,* which removes diseases of the legs. 55.

अथ मर्कटाशनम्[1] —
पादौ सम्पीड्य[2] हस्ताभ्यां अंगुष्ठौ[3] धारयेद् दृढम् ||
पादमध्ये शिरः क्षिप्त्वा धनुर्वन्मर्कटासनम्[4] || 56 ||

***atha markaṭāsanam* —**
pādau sampīḍya hastābhyāṃ aṅguṣṭhau dhārayed dṛḍham //
pādamadhye śiraḥ kṣiptvā dhanurvanmarkaṭāsanam // 56 //

Tr. Pressing the legs with the hands, firmly hold the big toes (from behind) and drop the head between the legs, imitating the form of a bow. This is *markaṭāsana.* 56.

अथ मत्स्येन्द्राशनम्[5] —
वामोरुमूलार्पितदक्षपादो[6] जान्वोर्बहिर्वेष्टितदक्षदोष्णा ||
प्रगृह्य तिष्ठेत्परिवर्तिताङ्गः श्रीमत्स्यनाथोदितमासनं स्यात् || 57 ||

***atha matsyendrāsanam* —**
vāmorumūlārpita dakṣapādo
jānvorbahirveṣṭitadakṣadoṣṇā //
pragṛhya tiṣṭhetparivartitāṅgaḥ
śrīmatsyanāthoditamāsanaṃ syāt // 57 //

Tr. Place the right foot at the root of the left thigh and place the left leg by the side of the right knee. Hold the left leg by the right hand and twist the body and remain steady. This *āsana* is propagated by *Matsyendranātha.* 57.

---

1. अथ कमठासनं –n2. 2. संस्थाप्य –n1. 3. अंगुष्ठे -P,T,t1. 4. कमठासनम् -n2.
5. मत्स्येन्द्रासन –J. 6. दक्षपादं-P, दक्षपादौ –t1.

मत्स्येन्द्रपीठं जठरप्रदीप्तं[1] प्रचण्डरुग्मण्डलखण्डनास्त्रम् ॥
अभ्यासतः कुण्डलिनीप्रबोधं दण्डस्थिरत्वं च ददाति पुंसाम् ॥ 58 ॥

matsyendrapīṭhaṃ jaṭharapradīptaṃ
pracaṇḍarugmaṇḍalakhaṇḍanāstram //
abhyāsataḥ kuṇḍalinīprabodhaṃ
daṇḍasthiratvaṃ ca dadāti puṃsām // 58 //

Tr. *Matsyendra-pīṭha* enhances the gastric fire and works like a weapon to destroy hosts of severe diseases. Moreover, it helps arousal of *kuṇḍalinī* and offers stability to the spine. 58.

Note: The technique of *matsyendrāsana* given here differs from the one available in GhS. In GhS (ii.22-23), the hand is bent in the elbow crossing the raised knee and the chin rests on the palm of the hand.

In the technique of *matsyendrāsana,* though only the left twist is described, it is to be repeated on the other side also giving the right twist, as suggested by *Brahmānanda*. 58.

पार्श्वाभ्यां ध्रियते यस्तु पार्श्वमत्स्येन्द्रमुत्तमम् ॥ 59 ॥

pārśvābhyāṃ dhriyate yastu pārśvamatsyendramuttamam/59/

Tr. When held by the sides, it forms *pārśva-matsyendra*, which is excellent. 59.

करेण बन्धयेत् तत्तु[2] बद्धमत्स्येन्द्रासनम्[3] ॥ 60 ॥

kareṇa bandhayet tattu baddhamatsyendrāsanam // 60 //

Tr. When tied with the hand, it makes *baddha-matsyendra*. 60.

Note: In these verses, two more varieties of *matsyendrāsana* are given, but the techniques are not clearly described. 59-60.

---

1. जठर प्रवृत्तं –T,t1, ज्वलनप्रवृत्तः -N,n1,n3,J. 2. तं तु –P,T,t1. 3. बद्धमत्स्येन्द्रमासनं –J,N,P.

अथ निरालम्बनम् —
कराभ्यां पंकजं कृत्वा तिष्ठेत्कूर्परया सुधीः ॥
मुखमुन्नमयन्नुच्चै[1]र्निरालम्बनमासनम् ॥ 61 ॥
atha nirālambanam —
karābhyāṃ paṅkajaṃ kṛtvā tiṣṭhetkūrparayā sudhīḥ //
mukhamunnamayanuccair nirālambanamāsanam // 61 //

Tr. Hands forming like a lotus and supporting on the elbows, raise the face up. This is called *nirālambanāsana*. 61.

निरालम्बनयोगी स्यान्निरालम्बनमासनम् ॥[2]
निरालम्बनता ध्यानं[3] निरालम्बनमासनम्[4] ॥ 62 ॥
nirālambanayogī syānnirālambanamāsanam //
nirālambanatā dhyānaṃ nirālambanamāsanam // 62 //

Tr. Practising *nirālambana āsana*, a *yogī* attains the state of *nirālambana*. The posture *nirālambana* culminates into *nirālambana dhyāna*. 62.

अथ सौरासनम्[5] —
प्रसार्यैकं पादतलं[6] संस्थाप्य त्वेकपादकम्[7] ॥ 63 ॥
atha saurāsanam —
prasāryaikaṃ pādatalaṃ saṃsthāpya tvekapādakam / 63/

Tr. Stretch out one leg and place the other foot on the ground. 63.

अथैकपादासनम्[8] —
एक[9]पादमथो कण्ठे उत्थाप्यैकं च दण्डवत् ॥
करौ सम्पुटितौ[10] कृत्वा एकपादं तदुच्यते ॥ 64 ॥
athaikapādāsanam —
ekapādamatho kaṇṭhe utthāpyaikaṃ ca daṇḍavat //
karau samputitau kṛtvā ekapādaṃ taducyate // 64 //

---

1. मुखमुन्नमयेच्च-N, सुखमुन्नमयन्नुच्चैः-T, मुखमुन्नमयन्नुच्च–J. 2. अनुपलब्धापंक्तिः-N,n1,n2,n3,J,t1. 3. शेषः-T. 4. अनुपलब्धपाठः-T. 5. अथ एकपादासनम्-T. 6. पादतले–J. 7. संस्थाप्यौकपादकम्-P. 8. एकपादासनम्-T. 9. एकं–P. 10. सम्पुटितं -N.

Tr. Having placed one leg over the neck, the other leg is raised up like a stick. The hands are folded on the chest. This is called *ekapāda*. 64.

अथ फणीन्द्रासनम्[1] —
पादाभ्यां वेष्टयेत्कण्ठं करयोः संस्थितोन्मुखम्[2] ॥
फणीन्द्रं सर्वदोषघ्नं वोभूयात्[3] सुखदं सदा ॥ 65 ॥[4]

atha phaṇīndrāsanam —
pādābhyāṃ veṣṭayetkaṇṭhaṃ karayoḥ saṃsthitonmukham //
phaṇīndraṃ sarvadoṣaghnaṃ vobhūyāt sukhadaṃ sadā //65 //

Tr. The neck is encircled with two legs and supporting (the body) with the hands, the face is turned upwards. This *phaṇīndra* removes all the ills and bestows upon one wellness for ever. 65.

अथ पश्चिमतानासनम्[5] —
प्रसार्य पादौ भुवि दण्डरूपौ दोर्भ्यां पदाग्र[6]द्वितयं गृहीत्वा[7] ॥
जानूपरि न्यस्तललाटदेशो वसेदिदं पश्चिमतानमाहुः ॥ 66 ॥[4]

atha paścimatānāsanam —
prasārya pādau bhuvi daṇḍarūpau
dorbhyāṃ padāgradvitayaṃ gṛhītvā //
jānūpari nyastalalāṭadeśo
vasedidaṃ paścimatānamāhuḥ // 66 //

Tr. Stretch both the legs on the ground. Hold the big toes by the respective hands and put the forehead on the knees. This forms *paścimatāna*. 66.

इति पश्चिमतानमासनाग्र्यं पवनं पश्चिमवाहिनं[8] करोति ॥
उदयं जठरानलस्य कुर्यादुदरे कार्श्यमरोगतां च पुंसाम् ॥ 67 ॥ [4]

1.फणीन्द्रम्-J,P,T. 2. संस्थितो मुनिः-P,T. 3. वाभूयात्-J. 4. अनुपलब्धश्लोकः -n2. 5.पश्चिमतानम्-J,P,T. 6. द्वाभ्यां कराभ्यां –n1,3. 7. द्वाभ्यां कराभ्यां द्वितयं गृहीत्वा-N,J. 8. वाहनं –J.

iti paścimatānamāsanāgryaṃ
pavanaṃ paścimavāhinaṃ karoti //
udayaṃ jaṭharānalasya kuryād
udare kārśyamarogatāṃ ca puṃsām // 67 //

Tr. *Paścimatāna* causes the currents of *prāṇa* to flow through *suṣumnā,* stimulates gastric fire, reduces the belly and brings good health to a person. 67.

Note: This is an important traditional *āsana*, which tones up nerves supplying the pelvic organs and arising from lumbo-sacral region. GhS(ii.26) calls it *paścimottānāsana.* ŚS (iii. 113-114) says that *ugrāsana* is a synonym for *paścimottānāsana,* although, there is a slight difference in the technique. 66-67.

शयितपश्चिमतानकम्[1] —
तानं शयित्वा[2] तु कुर्वीत शयितपश्चिमतानकम्[3] ‖ 68 ‖ *
***śayitapaścimatānakam* —**
tānaṃ śayitvā tu kurvīta śayitapaścimatānakam // 68 //

Tr. Lie supine and practise *paścimatāna* to form *śayita-paścimatāna.* 68.

Note: For discussion on the varieties of *paścimatāna*, see YM (vol. 20, No. 4, pp. 56-66). 68.

अथ विचित्रकरणीनामासनम्[4] —
शयितपश्चिमतानस्थे[5] हस्तौ[6] तत्र[7] प्रसारयेत् ‖
पादौ दण्डसमौ कृत्वा[8] विचित्रकरणी भवेत् ‖ 69 ‖*
***atha vicitrakaraṇīnāmāsanam* —**
śayitapaścimatānasthe hastau tatra prasārayet //
pādau daṇḍasamau kṛtvā vicitrakaraṇī bhavet // 69 //

Tr. Adopting *śayita-paścimatāna,* extend the hands and straighten the legs like stick. This is *vicitra-karaṇī.* 69.

---

1 . शयितताणम्-P, शयितासनम् -N,n1; शेशे ताणं-T; शयीनासनम्-J. 2 . शेत्वा-P, ताणे शेत्वा-T. 3 . शैत- पश्चिमाताणकं-T; सैवपश्चिमताणकम्-N,J. 4 . विचित्रीनामासनं-J. 5 . शतपाश्चिमतारस्थः-J,N. 6 . करौ-P,T,t1,.7 . तत्-P,T,t1. 8 . कार्यौ -P,T,t1.
* अनुपलब्धश्लोकः-n2,n3.

अथ योगनिद्रासनम्[1] —

पादाभ्यां वेष्टयेत्कण्ठं हस्ताभ्यां पृष्ठबन्धनम् ||
तन्मध्ये शयनं कुर्याद् योगनिद्रा सुखप्रदा || 70 ||

atha yoganidrāsanam —
pādābhyāṃ veṣṭayetkaṇṭhaṃ hastābhyāṃ pṛṣṭhabandhanam /
tanmadhye śayanaṃ kuryād yoganidrā sukhapradā // 70 //

Tr. Wind the legs around the neck, tie up the hands on the back and lie down. This is *yoganidrā,* which offers wellbeing. 70.

अथ विधूननम्[2] —

गुल्फ[3]स्थितौ पादमेकं प्रसार्य
तत्पादाग्रं संस्पृशेत्तत्करेण[4] ||
गुल्फं चान्यं धारयेत्तत्करेण
धूनं पीठं चाभ्यसेच्चोभयत्र || 71 ||

atha vidhūnanam —
gulphasthitau pādamekaṃ prasārya
tatpādāgraṃ saṃspṛśettatkareṇa //
gulphaṃ cānyaṃ dhārayettatkareṇa
dhūnaṃ pīṭhaṃ cābhyaseccobhayatra // 71 //

Tr. Resting on one heel, stretch the other leg and touch its toes with the respective hand. The other heel is held with the other hand. This is *dhūna-pīṭha,* which should be practised on both the sides. 71.

अथ पादपीडनासनम्[5] —

स्थित्वैकस्मिन् पादतले कराभ्यां वेष्टयेत्तनुम् ||
पृष्ठे संस्थाप्य यत्नेन पादपीडनमासनम्[6] || 72 ||

atha pādapīḍanāsanam —
sthitvaikasmin pādatale karābhyāṃ veṣṭayettanum //
pṛṣṭhe saṃsthāpya yatnena pādapīḍanamāsanam // 72 //

---

1. अथ योगनिद्रा –J,P,T, अनुपलब्धपंक्तिः-n2,n3 . 2. अथ विधूनासनम् -N,n1. 3 . गुल्फौ -P,T,t1. 4. पादौ –J,N,T. 5 . पादपीठासनम् -P,T,n1,n2. 6 . पादपीठनमासनम्-P,T,t1.

Tr. Stand on one leg. Fold the other leg at the back and hold it with the hands. This is called *pādapīḍanāsana*. 72.

अथ कुक्कुटासनम् —

पद्मासनं सुसंस्थाप्य[1] जानूर्वोरन्तरे करौ[2] ॥
निवेश्य भूमौ संस्थाप्य व्योमस्थः[3] कुक्कुटासनम् ॥ 73 ॥

atha kukkuṭāsanam —

padmāsanaṃ susaṃsthāpya jānūrvorantare karau //
niveśya bhūmau saṃsthāpya vyomasthaḥ kukkuṭāsanam /73/

Tr. Adopt *padmāsana*, insert the arms between the knees and the thighs and firmly place the palms on the ground and remain aloft. This is known as *kukkuṭāsana*. 73.

Note: *Śrīnivāsa* mentions five varieties of *kukkuṭāsana*, namely, *pañcaculī-kukkuṭa, ekapāda-kukkuṭa, ākārita-kukkuṭa, bandhaculī-kukkuṭa* and *pārśva-kukkuṭa*, but does not describe them. In this verse, he describes only one variety, but which is this variety, is not clear. KKHP describes *paṅgu-kukkuṭāsana*, where the foot-lock is raised by balancing on one hand, the other hand grasping the wrist of the balancing hand. 73.

अथोत्तानकूर्मासनम्[4] —

कुक्कुटासनबन्धस्थो दोर्भ्यां सम्बध्य कन्धराम्[5] ॥
शेते कूर्मवदुत्तानमेतदुत्तानकूर्मकम्[6] ॥ 74 ॥

athottānakūrmāsanam —

kukkuṭāsanabandhastho dorbhyāṃ saṃbadhya kandharām //
śete kūrmavaduttānametaduttānakūrmakam // 74 //

Tr. Assume *kukkuṭāsana*, wind the arms around the neck and lie on the back like a tortoise. This is *uttāna-kūrmāsana*. 74.

Note: *Nārāyaṇatīrtha* in YSC(ii.46-{12}) calls it *uttāna-kukkuṭāsana*. 74.

---

1. सुखं स्थाप्य –N,n1. 2. तथा –P,T,t1. 3. व्योमस्थ –J, व्योमस्थं –P,t1. 4. अथोत्तानकूर्मकम् -T, अथोत्तानकूर्म -n2. 5. कन्धरम् -N,n2, कन्दरम् -T. 6. एतदुत्थानकूर्मकम् T, कूर्मके –J.

अथ वृश्चिकासनम् —

हस्तौ[1] धरामवष्टभ्य चरणौ भालसंस्थितौ[2] ॥
गुल्फौ स्यातामुन्मुखः सन् वृश्चिकासनमीर्यते ॥ 75 ॥

atha vṛścikāsanam —

hastau dharāmavaṣṭabhya caraṇau bhālasaṃsthitau //
gulphau syātāmunmukhaḥ san vṛścikāsanamīryate // 75 //

Tr. Fix the hands on the ground, place the feet on the forehead, keeping the heels upturned. This is called *vṛścikāsana.* 75.

ग्रन्थविस्तारभीत्या तु सर्वेषां च न लक्षितम्[3] ॥

granthavistārabhītyā tu sarveṣāṃ ca na lakṣitam //

Tr. All the *āsanas* are not described due to the apprehension that it may inflate the size of the book.

अथान्तिमं शवासनम्[4] —

प्रसार्य हस्तपादौ[5] च विश्रान्त्या शयनं तथा ॥
सर्वासन[6]श्रमहरं शयितं तु शवासनम् ॥ 76 ॥

इत्यासननिरूपणम्[7] ॥

athāntimaṃ śavāsanam —

prasārya hastapādau ca viśrāntyā śayanaṃ tathā //
sarvāsanaśramaharaṃ śayitaṃ tu śavāsanam // 76 //

ityāsananirūpaṇam //

Lastly *śavāsana*—

Tr. Spread out the hands and legs, while lying relaxed. *śavāsana*, which is practised in lying position, relieves fatigue caused due to practice of (all the) *āsanas*. 76.

Thus ends the description of *āsanas*.

---

1. पादौ –J,N,n1,n2,n3,T,t1. 2. फालसंस्थितौ –P,T,t1. 3. सर्वेषान्नचलक्षणम् -N,n3,J. 4. अन्तिमं शवासनम् -N. 5. हस्तौ पादौ -P,T,t1. 6. सवासन -J,N,n1. 7. अनुपलब्धपंक्तिः -T.

आसनेन रुजं हन्ति प्राणायामेन पातकम् ॥
प्रत्याहारेण योगीन्द्रो विकारं हन्ति मानसम् ॥ 77 ॥
āsanena rujaṃ hanti prāṇāyāmena pātakam //
pratyāhāreṇa yogīndro vikāraṃ hanti mānasam // 77 //

Tr. *Āsanas* alleviate diseases, *prāṇāyāma* removes the sins and practice of *pratyāhāra* brings an end to mental ills of a *yogī*. 77.

Note: The sequence of verse No. 76 and 77 has been changed by the Editors to suit the proper presentation of the text. 77.

अथ प्राणायामः[1] —
अथासने दृढे योगी वशी हितमिताशनः[2] ॥
गुरूपदिष्टमार्गेण प्राणायामान्[3] समभ्यसेत् ॥ 78 ॥
atha prāṇāyāmaḥ —
athāsane dṛḍhe yogī vaśī hitamitāśanaḥ //
gurūpadiṣṭamārgeṇa prāṇāyāmān samabhyaset // 78 //

Tr. Having attained perfection in *āsana*, a *yogī*, who is self-restrained and who consumes wholesome and moderate food, should undertake the practice of *prāṇāyāma*, as instructed by the *guru*. 78.

[4]चले वाते चलं चित्तं[5] निश्चले[6] निश्चलं तथा[7] ॥ [8]
योगी स्थाणुत्वमाप्नोति ततो वायुं निरुन्धयेत्[9] ॥ 79 ॥
cale vāte calaṃ cittaṃ niścale niścalaṃ tathā //
yogī sthāṇutvamāpnoti tato vāyuṃ nirundhayet // 79 //

Tr. Mind becomes unstable as the breathing increases. When breathing is controlled, mind becomes stable and a *yogī* attains steadiness. Therefore the *vāyu* should be restrained. 79.

यावद्वायुः स्थितो देहे तावज्जीवितमुच्यते ॥
मरणं तस्य निष्क्रान्ति[10]स्ततो वायुं निरोधयेत्[11] ॥ 80 ॥

---

1. अथ प्राणायामप्रकरणं –n3. 2. मितहिताशनः-J. 3. प्राणायामं –n2. 4. अथ दृढबन्धनम्-अधिकपाठः -N,P. 5 . सर्व-P,T,t1, बिन्दु-n2. 6 . निश्चिते-P; अनुपलब्ध-T. 7 . तथा-N, निश्चलं तथा-J,n1, निश्चलं भवेत-n3. हठबन्धनम्-P,n1,n2,t1. 8. दृढबन्धनम्-अधिकपाठः-P, इत्यासननिरूपणम्- अधिकपाठः-T,t1. 9. वायुनिबन्धनात्-P,T,t1, निबन्धयेत्-n2. 10. निष्क्रान्ते–P,T,t1. 11 . निरुन्धयेत्-N,n1,n3,J.

yāvadvāyuḥ sthito dehe tāvajjīvitamucyate //
maraṇaṃ tasya niṣkrāntistato vāyuṃ nirodhayet // 80 //

Tr. Life exists so long as the *vāyu* (*prāṇa*) remains in the body. Death means the exit of *prāṇa*. Therefore, *prāṇa* should be controlled. 80.

मलाकुलासु नाडीषु मारुतो नैव मध्यगः ॥
कथं स्यादुन्मनीभावः कायसिद्धिः[1] कथं भवेत् ॥ 81 ॥ *
malākulāsu nāḍīṣu māruto naiva madhyagaḥ //
kathaṃ syādunmanībhāvaḥ kāyasiddhiḥ kathaṃ bhavet /81/

Tr. The *māruta* (*prāṇa*) cannot freely pass through the middle *nāḍī* (*suṣumnā*) due to morbidities in it. How can then one attain *unmanī* state and supernormal bodily powers. 81.

ब्रह्मादयोऽपि त्रिदशाः पवनाभ्यासतत्पराः ॥
अभूवन्मृत्युरहिता[2]स्तस्मात्पवनमभ्यसेत् ॥ 82 ॥
brahmādayo'pi tridaśāḥ pavanābhyāsatatparāḥ //
abhūvanmṛtyurahitāstasmātpavanamabhyaset // 82 //

Tr. Even the gods like *Brahmā* etc. became free from death through consistent practice of *prāṇāyāma*. Therefore, one should practise *prāṇāyāma*. 82.

[3]सिद्धे वा बद्धपद्मे वा स्वस्तिके चाथवासने[4] ॥
ऋजुकायः समासीनः प्राणायामान्समभ्यसेत् ॥ 83 ॥ *
siddhe vā baddhapadme vā svastike cāthavāsane //
ṛjukāyaḥ samāsīnaḥ prāṇāyāmānsamabhyaset // 83 //

Tr. Adopt *siddha, baddha-padma* or *svastikāsana* and keeping the body erect, practise *prāṇāyāma*. 83.

---

1 . **कार्यसिद्धिः**-J,N,t1. 2 . **अभूवन्नन्तकभयात्त**-P,T,t1. 3. **अथ प्राणायामप्रकार**-P,T, **अथ प्राणायामः** -n2. 4. **वा भवासने**–P, **वाथवासने**–T,t1,n1. * **अनुपलब्धश्लोकः** -n3.

पद्मासनस्थितो योगी प्राणं चन्द्रेण पूरयेत् ||[1]
प्राणं सूर्येण[2] चाकृष्य पूरयित्वोदरं शनैः || 84 ||
विधिवत्कुम्भकं कृत्वा पुनश्चन्द्रेण रेचयेत् ||
येन त्यजेत्तेनापूर्य[3] धारयेदविरोधतः[4] || 85 ||[5]

padmāsanasthito yogī prāṇaṃ candreṇa pūrayet //
prāṇaṃ sūryeṇa cākṛṣya pūrayitvodaraṃ śanaiḥ // 84 //
vidhivatkumbhakaṃ kṛtvā punaścandreṇa recayet //
yena tyajettenāpūrya dhārayedavirodhataḥ // 85 //

Tr. Sit in *padmāsana*, draw *prāna* in through *candra* (left nostril) {See note}. Gently draw the *prāṇa* through *sūrya* (right nostril) and fill up the cavity. Retain the air in the prescribed manner and exhale through *candra* (left nostril). Inhale through the same nostril, through which exhalation is done and comfortably hold the breath. 84-85.

Note: After the first line, the next line seems to be missing. HP-iv.11 (10 chapters) properly gives this missing line as "**धारयित्वा यथाशक्ति पुनः सूर्येण रेचयेत्**", which means, "one should exhale through the *sūryanāḍī* (right nostril) after holding the breath to the capacity". 84-85.

प्राणं चेदिडया पिबेन्नियमितं[6] भूयोऽन्यया[7] रेचयेत्
पीत्वा पिंगलया समीरणमथो बद्ध्वा[8] त्यजेद्वामया[9] ||
सूर्याचन्द्रमसोरनेन विधिना बिम्बद्वयं ध्यायताम्
शुद्धा नाडिगणा[10] भवन्ति यमिनां मासत्रयादूर्ध्वतः || 86 ||

prāṇaṃ cediḍayā pibenniyamitaṃ bhūyo'nyayā recayet
pītvā piṅgalayā samīraṇamatho baddhvā tyajedvāmayā//
sūryācandramasoranena vidhinā bimbadvayaṃ dhyāyatām
śuddhā nāḍigaṇā bhavanti yamināṃ māsatrayādūrdhvataḥ 86

Tr. Regularly inhale *prāṇa* through *iḍā* and exhale through the other. Thereafter, draw the air in through *piṅgalā*, retain and

---

1. येन त्यजेत्तेन पूर्य धारयेदनिरोधतः- अधिकः पाठः -P,T,t1. 2. चन्द्रेण-N. 3. त्यजेत्तेन सूर्य-J, तेन पूर्य ˙ –P. 4. धारयेदनिरोधतः-P. 5. अनुपलब्धः-P,T,t1. 6. परिमितं –n3. 7. भूयोऽन्यथा–J,T. 8. बद्धं-N,n1,J. 9. त्येजेन्प्राप्नुयात्-P,T,t1. 10. नाडीगणा–P.

exhale through the left (nostril). This practice is done through *sūrya* and *candra,* while visualizing the two discs (of the Sun and Moon). The *yogīs* attain purification of the group of the *nāḍīs* after three months. 86.

Note: The term '*bimbadvaya*' refers to two disks of the sun and moon. 86.

प्रातर्मध्यन्दिने सायमर्धरात्रे[1] च कुम्भकान् ॥
शनैरशीतिपर्यन्तं चतुर्वारं समभ्यसेत् ॥ 87 ॥
prātarmadhyandine sāyamardharātre ca kumbhakān //
śanairaśītiparyantaṃ caturvāraṃ samabhyaset // 87 //

Tr. One should practise eighty rounds of *kumbhakas* increasing gradually four times in a day, in the morning, noon, evening and midnight. 87.

कनीयसि भवेत्स्वेदः कम्पो भवति मध्यमे ॥
उत्तिष्ठत्युत्तमे[2] प्राणरोधे पद्मासने[3] मुहुः ॥ 88 ॥
kanīyasi bhavetsvedaḥ kampo bhavati madhyame //
uttiṣṭhatyuttame prāṇarodhe padmāsane muhuḥ // 88 //

Tr. Lower type of *prāṇāyāma* generates perspiration, medium one causes tremors, while one levitates during the practice of superior type of *prāṇāyāma* when adopting *padmāsana*. 88.

जलेन श्रमजातेन अङ्गमर्दनमाचरेत् ॥
दृढता लघुता चापि तथा गात्रस्य जायते ॥ 89 ॥[4]
jalena śramajātena aṅgamardanamācaret //
dṛḍhatā laghutā cāpi tathā gātrasya jāyate // 89 //

Tr. One will do well by rubbing the body with the sweat generated by exertion (of *prāṇāyāma*). This makes the body strong and light. 89.

---

1. मर्द्धरात्रौ–J,N. 2. उत्तिष्ठेदुत्तमे-P,T. 3. पद्मासनं-P,T,t1. 4. अनुपलब्धः-T,t1,N,n1,n2,n3,J.

यथा सिंहो गजो व्याघ्रो भवेद्वश्यः[1] शनैः शनैः ॥
तथैव सेवितो वायुर्भवेद्वश्यः[1] शनैः शनैः[2] ॥ 90 ॥
yathā siṃho gajo vyāghro bhavedvaśyaḥ śanaiḥ śanaiḥ //
tathaiva sevito vāyurbhavedvaśyaḥ śanaiḥ śanaiḥ // 90 //

Tr. As one can gradually tame a lion, an elephant or a tiger, similarly, *prāṇa* must be controlled slowly through a gradual practice. 90.

प्राणायामेन युक्तेन सर्वरोगक्षयो भवेत्
अयुक्ताभ्यासयोगेन सर्वरोगसमुद्भवः ॥ 91 ॥[3]
हिक्का[4] श्वासश्च[5] कासश्च शिरःकर्णाक्षिवेदनाः ॥
भवन्ति विविधा रोगाः पवनस्य व्यतिक्रमात् ॥ 92 ॥
prāṇāyāmena yuktena sarvarogakṣayo bhavet //
ayuktābhyāsayogena sarvarogasamudbhavaḥ // 91 //
hikkā śvāsaśca kāsaśca śiraḥkarṇākṣivedanāḥ //
bhavanti vividhā rogāḥ pavanasya vyatikramāt // 92 //

Tr. Proper practice of *prāṇāyāma* alleviates all the diseases, whereas improper practice of *prāṇāyāma* invites all the disorders. An incorrect practice of *prāṇāyāma* causes several disorders, like—hiccup, cough, asthma and pain in the head, ears and eyes. 91-92.

युक्तं युक्तं त्यजेद्वायुं युक्तं युक्तं प्रपूरयेत्[6] ॥
युक्तं युक्तं च बध्नीयादेवं सिद्धिमवाप्नुयात् ॥ 93 ॥
yuktaṃ yuktaṃ tyajedvāyuṃ yuktaṃ yuktaṃ prapūrayet //
yuktaṃ yuktaṃ ca badhnīyādevaṃ siddhimavāpnuyāt // 93 //

Tr. To get success, one should inhale, retain and exhale in a very judicious and controlled manner. 93.

यदा तु नाडीशुद्धिः स्यात् तदा चिह्नानि बाह्यतः ॥
कायस्य कृशता कान्तिर्जायते तस्य निश्चितम्[7] ॥ 94 ॥

---

1. वश्यं–J,N. 2. ...वायुरन्यथा हन्ति साधकः-P,T,t1, अनुपलब्धपंक्तिः -n2.. 3. अनुपलब्धश्लोकः-J,N,n1,n2,n3. 4. वायुः-N,n1,n3,J. 5. भ्यासश्च -T. 6. च पूरयेत् -P,T,t1. 7. कान्तिस्तथा जायेत निश्चितं -P,T,t1.

yadā tu nāḍīśuddhiḥ syāt tadā cihnāni bāhyataḥ //
kāyasya kṛśatā kāntirjāyate tasya niścitam // 94 //

Tr. When the *nāḍīs* are purified, the external signs certainly seen are – slimness and lustre of the body. 94.

यथेष्टं धारणं वायोरनलस्य प्रदीपनम् ॥
नादाभिव्यक्तिरारोग्यं जायते नाडिशोधनात् ॥ 95 ॥
yatheṣṭaṃ dhāraṇaṃ vāyoranalasya pradīpanam //
nādābhivyaktirārogyaṃ jāyate nāḍiśodhanāt // 95 //

Tr. As a result of purification of the *nāḍīs*, one is able to retain the breath longer, (one enjoys) increase in (bodily) fire, manifestation of the internally aroused sound and feeling of well-being. 95.

योगी[1] याज्ञवल्क्येनोक्तम् —
सव्याहृतिं[2] सप्रणवां गायत्रीं शिरसा सह ॥
त्रिः पठेदायतः प्राणः प्राणायामः स उच्यते ॥ 96 ॥

yogī yājñavalkyenoktam —
savyāhṛtiṃ sapraṇavāṃ gāyatrīṃ śirasā saha //
triḥ paṭhedāyataḥ prāṇaḥ prāṇāyāmaḥ sa ucyate // 96 //

According to *Yogī Yājñavalkya*—

Tr. During the retention of breath, recite *gāyatrī* for three times alongwith *vyāhṛtis, praṇava* and *śiras*. This is called *prāṇāyāma*. 96.

Note: The technique of *prāṇāyāma* described in this verse refers to the *smārta prāṇāyāma*, in which the *prāṇāyāma* is accompanied with the recitation of *om* (*praṇava*), *vyāhṛti*, *gāyatrī* and *śiras*. 96.

---

1. योगि -P,J, योगयाज्ञवल्क्याचार्यैरुक्तम्-T. 2. सव्याहृतीं –P,T.

अत्र शिववचनम् —
प्राणायामपरो योगी सोऽपि विष्णुर्महेश्वरः ॥
सर्वदेवमयो योगी तस्यावज्ञां न कारयेत् ॥ 97 ॥
इति प्राणायामनिरूपणम्[1] ॥

atra śivavacanam —
prāṇāyāmaparo yogī so'pi viṣṇurmaheśvaraḥ //
sarvadevamayo yogī tasyāvajñāṃ na kārayet // 97 //
iti prāṇāyāmanirūpaṇam *//*

According to *Siva*—

Tr. A *yogī,* who is devoted to the practice of *prāṇāyāma* is like *Viṣṇu* and *Maheśvara.* Such a *yogī* is a representation of all the gods. One should not disrespect such a *yogī.* 97.

Thus ends the description of *prāṇāyāma.*

[2]इति श्रीनिवासयोगीविरचितायां[3] हठरत्नावल्यां तृतीयोपदेशः[4]

iti śrīnivāsayogīviracitāyāṃ haṭharatnāvalyāṃ tṛtīyopadeśaḥ

Here ends the third chapter of haṭharatnāvalī composed by yogī Śrīnivāsa

---

1. इति प्राणायामनियमः -n2.
2. इति श्रीनिवासयोगीश्वरविरचितायाम् -n2.
नानास्वस्तिकसिद्धपद्मकमहावीरासनाद्यान्वितः
प्राणायामसमन्वितश्च ललितः श्रीश्रीनिवासोदितः ॥
ख्याते रम्यसुवर्णराजखचिते रत्नावलीनामके
ग्रन्थेऽस्मिन्नुपदेश एष विहितारम्भस्तृतीयो गतः ॥ अधिकः पाठः-P,T.
3. इति श्रीनिवासयोगीन्द्रविरचितायां-P,T.
4. इति हठरत्नावल्यां तृतीयोपदेशः-J,n3.

हठरत्नावली

चतुर्थोपदेशः

अत्र समाधिः[1] —
सलिले सैन्धवं यद्वत् साम्यं भवति योगवित् ॥
तथात्ममनसोरैक्यं[2] समाधिः सोऽभिधीयते ॥ 1 ॥

***atra samādhiḥ* —**
salile saindhavaṃ yadvat sāmyaṃ bhavati yogavit //
tathātmamanasoraikyaṃ samādhiḥ so'bhidhīyate // 1 //

Tr. As salt is dissolved in water, likewise, a learned *yogī* attains unity of soul and mind. This is called *samādhi*. 1

मतान्तरेऽपि[3] —
तत्समत्वं भवेदत्र जीवात्मपरमात्मनोः ॥
समस्तनष्टसंकल्पः[4] समाधिः सोऽभिधीयते ॥ 2 ॥

***matāntare'pi* —**
tatsamatvaṃ bhavedatra jīvātmaparamātmanoḥ //
samastanaṣṭasaṅkalpaḥ samādhiḥ so'bhidhīyate // 2 //

Another opinion—

Tr. Union of *Jīvātmā* and *Paramātmā* eliminates all mental constructions. This is called *samādhi*. 2.

ध्यानादस्पन्दमनसः समाधिः सोऽभिधीयते ॥ 3 ॥
dhyānādaspandamanasaḥ samādhiḥ so'bhidhīyate // 3 //

Tr. In the state of *dhyāna*, mind becomes steady. This is called *samādhi*. 3.

अतिविस्तारभीत्या[5] तु न सर्वमिह लिख्यते ॥
ativistārabhītyā tu na sarvamiha likhyate //

---

1. अनुपलब्धः -N,n1,n2,n3,J. 2. तथातन्मनसोरैक्यं-N,J. 3. अनुपलब्धपंक्तिः-n2.
4. समस्तनष्टसंकल्पं -J. 5. अतिविस्तारवृत्या-J; अविस्तारवृत्या-N,n1.

Tr. Details are avoided, for the fear of great elaboration.

इन्द्रियाणां मनो नाथो मनोनाथस्तु मारुतः ॥
मारुतस्य लयो नाथः[1] स लयो नादमाश्रितः[2] ॥ 4 ॥
indriyāṇām mano nātho manonāthastu mārutaḥ //
mārutasya layo nāthaḥ sa layo nādamāśritaḥ //4 //

Tr. Mind is the lord of the senses, *māruta* (*prāṇa*) is the lord of the mind, while *laya* is the lord of *māruta* and that *laya* is sustained by *nāda* (sound). 4.

Note: This verse seems to have been taken from HP (iv.29), where we get the reading '*sa layo nādamāśritaḥ*'. Although this reading is not available in any of the Mss, we have adopted it, since it is more appropriate. 4.

अथ नादानुसन्धानम् —
नादानुसन्धानसमाधिभाजां
योगीश्वराणां हृदये प्ररूढम् ॥
आनन्दमेकं[3] वचसोऽप्यगम्यं[4]
जानाति तं श्रीगुरुनाथ एव[5] ॥ 5 ॥
atha nādānusandhānam —
nādānusandhānasamādhibhājām
yogīśvarāṇām hṛdaye prarūḍham //
ānandamekam vacaso'pyagamyam
jānāti tam śrīgurunātha eva // 5 //

Tr. The great *yogīs*, who experience the state of *samādhi* by meditating on *nāda*, experience an inexplicable joy in their heart, which only *Śrī Gurunātha* knows. 5.

उदासीनपरो भूत्वा सदाभ्यासेन संयमी ॥
उन्मनीकरणं[6] सद्यो नादमेवावधारयेत्[7] ॥ 6 ॥

---

1. नादः-P,T,t1 नाथो–n2. 2. तन्नाथं-N,n2,J, तन्नादं लयमाश्रयेत्-P,T,n1, नाथस्तस्मात्तं–n3. 3. अनन्तमेकं-P,T,t1. 4. वचसामगम्यं-P,T,t1. 5. श्रीगुरुनाथमेकं–n2. 6. उन्मनी कारणं–P. 7. नादमेवानुधारयेत् -P,T,t1.

udāsīnaparo bhūtvā sadābhyāsena saṃyamī //
unmanīkaraṇaṃ sadyo nādamevāvadhārayet // 6 //

Tr. Through constant practice, being indifferent and with restraint, a *yogī* should take recourse to *nāda* alone, which instantly brings about the state of *unmanī*. 6.

शीते काले द्वौ पटी वा पटी वा[1]
पथ्याहारे गोपयो[2] वा पयो वा ॥
भक्ष्ये भोज्ये[3] वृत्तिमारण्यकं वा[4]
पाणी[5] द्रोणी कोऽपि[6] वा भक्ष्यपात्रे [7] ॥ 7 ॥

śīte kāle dvau paṭī vā paṭī vā
pathyāhāre gopayo vā payo vā //
bhakṣye bhojye vṛttimāraṇyakaṃ vā
pāṇī droṇī ko'pi vā bhakṣyapātre // 7 //

Tr. In the winter season, one may wear a single sheet of cloth or a folded one, he may consume cow milk or water, he may subsist on alms or on roots available in the forest, he may eat in the hands or in any (vessel) plate. 7.

कर्णौ पिधाय तूलेन[8] यः शृणोति[9] ध्वनिं यमी[10] ॥
तत्र चित्तं स्थिरं[11] कुर्याद्यावत् स्थिरपदं व्रजेत् ॥ 8 ॥

karṇau pidhāya tūlena yaḥ śṛṇoti dhvaniṃ yamī //
tatra cittaṃ sthiraṃ kuryādyāvat sthirapadaṃ vrajet // 8 //

Tr. A *yogī* plugs the ears with cotton and listens to the sound (*nāda*). He should focus the mind on that (*nāda*) till he attains steadiness of mind. 8.

श्रूयते[12] प्रथमाभ्यासे नादो नानाविधो बहुः[13] ॥
वर्धमाने ततोऽभ्यासे श्रूयते सूक्ष्मसूक्ष्मतः ॥ 9 ॥

śrūyate prathamābhyāse nādo nānāvidho bahuḥ //
vardhamāne tato'bhyāse śrūyate sūkṣmasūkṣmataḥ // 9 //

---

1. कुटी वा-T,t1. 2. गोमयो–J. 3. भोज्ये भक्ष्ये–P,t1. 4. वृंत्तमारण्यकं वा-P,n1. 5. पाणि–J,N,n1. 6. द्रोणीपि–J, कापि–N,n1. 7. भोज्यपत्रे–P,T,t1. 8. मूलेन-P,T,t1. 9. यं शृणोति–P, संशृणोति–N, n1,n2,n3,n4. 10. मुनिः-P,T. 11. स्थिरी-P. 12. श्रूयतां–T,t1. 13. बहून्-T,n2, बहु–J,n1, नादान्नानाविधान् बहून्-P,T,t1.

Tr. In the initial stages various sounds are heard. As one progresses, subtle and subtler sounds are heard. 9.

आदौ जलधिजीमूतभेरीनिर्झरसम्भवाः[1] ॥
मध्ये मर्द्दलशंखोत्था घण्टाकाहलकास्तथा[2] ॥ 10 ॥
अन्ते[3] तु किंकिणीवृन्द[4]वीणाभ्रमरनिःस्वनाः ॥
इति नानाविधा नादाः श्रूयन्ते देहमध्यतः ॥ 11 ॥
ādau jaladhijīmūtabherīnirjharasaṃbhavāḥ //
madhye marddalaśaṅkhotthā ghaṇṭākāhalakāstathā // 10 //
ante tu kiṅkiṇīvṛndavīṇābhramaraniḥsvanāḥ //
iti nānāvidhā nādāḥ śrūyante dehamadhyataḥ // 11 //

Tr. In the beginning, sounds resembling those of the ocean, thunder, big drum and waterfall are heard. In the intermediate stage, sounds like those of small drum, conch, bell and gong are heard. While in the end, sounds like those of tiny bells, *vīṇā* and humming of bees are heard. Thus, various sounds are heard within the body. 10-11.

मकरन्दं पिबेद् भृंगो गन्धो न प्रेक्ष्यते यथा[5] ॥
नादासक्तं तथा चित्तं विषयान्नहि[6] कांक्षते ॥ 12 ॥
makarandaṃ pibedbhṛṅgo gandho na prekṣyate yathā //
nādāsaktaṃ tathā cittaṃ viṣayānnahi kāṅkṣate // 12 //

Tr. A bee who enjoys the nectar, would not care for fragrance. In the same manner, the mind having been absorbed in *nāda*, would not run after the objects. 12.

सर्वचिन्तां[7] समुत्सृज्य सर्वचेष्टां च सर्वदा ॥
नादमेवानुसन्धानान्नादे[8] चित्तं विलीयते ॥ 13 ॥
sarvacintāṃ samutsṛjya sarvaceṣṭāṃ ca sarvadā //
nādamevānusandhānānnāde cittaṃ vilīyate // 13 //

Tr. On giving up all the thoughts and all the efforts, while always following the *nāda*, the *citta* merges into *nāda*. 13.

---

1. सन्निभाः-n3. 2. घण्टाकाहालकास्तथा-N,n1,J. 3. अन्ये-P; अन्त्ये-T,t1. 4. वंश–P.
5. गन्धान्नापेक्ष्यते यथा–n3, गंधानपि पिबेत्तथा-P,t1; (लुप्त) न्नपि पिबेत्तथा -T.
6. विषया न हि -J. 7. सर्व चिन्त्यं -P,T, सर्वचित्तं–J,N,n1. 8. नादमेवानुसंदध्यान्नादे-P.

सर्वचिन्तां[1] परित्यज्य सावधानेन चेतसा ॥
नाद एवानुसन्धेयः[2] योगसाम्राज्यसिद्धये[3] ॥ 14 ॥
sarvacintāṃ parityajya sāvadhānena cetasā //
nāda evānusandheyaḥ yogasāmrājyasiddhaye // 14 //

Tr. To attain the kingdom of *yoga*, one should relinquish all thoughts and carefully follow *nāda* alone. 14.

काष्ठे प्रवर्तितो वह्निः काष्ठेन सह लीयते ॥
नादे प्रवर्त्तितं चित्तं नादेन सह शाम्यति ॥ 15 ॥
kāṣṭhe pravartito vahniḥ kāṣṭhena saha līyate //
nāde pravartitaṃ cittaṃ nādena saha śāmyati // 15 //

Tr. Just as fire in the burning wood extinguishes alongwith the wood, similarly, *citta,* which is concentrated on *nāda*, merges with *nāda* itself. 15.

अस्तु वा मास्तु वा मुक्तिरत्रैवाखण्डितं महत् ॥
लयामृतं लये सौख्यं[4] राजयोगादवाप्यते ॥ 16 ॥
astu vā māstu vā muktiratraivākhaṇḍitaṃ mahat //
layāmṛtaṃ laye saukhyaṃ rājayogādavāpyate // 16 //

Tr. There might be or might not be a state of liberation, but this certainly is the state of profound and uninterrupted Bliss. This Blissful state of absorption is attained through *rājayoga*. 16.

अथ योगावस्था[5] —
आरम्भश्च घटश्चैव तथा परिचयस्तथा[6] ॥
निष्पत्तिः[7] सर्वयोगेषु योगावस्था भवन्ति ताः ॥ 17 ॥
***atha yogāvasthā* —**
ārambhaśca ghaṭaścaiva tathā paricayastathā /
niṣpattiḥ sarvayogeṣu yogāvasthā bhavanti tāḥ // 17 //

Tr. *Ārambha, ghaṭa, paricaya* and *niṣpatti* are the states of *yoga* described in all the (traditions of) *yoga*. 17.

---

1. सर्वचित्तं–T, सर्वचिन्त्यं –t1. 2. नादो यैरनुसंधेयो-N,n1,J, नाद एवानुसन्धेयाः-T. 3. योगसाम्राज्यमिच्छता-P,T. 4. सांख्यं -N,J, लयामृतलये सौख्यं–n1. 5. अनुपलब्धपंक्तिः-J. 6. ततः -n3. 7. निवृत्तिः-N,n1,n2,J.

ब्रह्मरन्ध्रे[1] भवेद् भेदो यो नादः[2] सूर्यसम्भवः ॥
विचित्रक्वणदो[3] देहेऽनाहतः श्रूयते ध्वनिः[4] ॥ 18 ॥
दिव्यदेहः सुतेजस्वी दिव्यगन्धस्त्वरोगवान्[5] ॥
सम्पूर्णहृदये[6] शून्ये त्वारम्भे योगवान् भवेत् ॥ 19 ॥

brahmarandhre bhavedbhedo yo nādaḥ sūryasambhavaḥ //
vicitrakvaṇado dehe'nāhataḥ śrūyate dhvaniḥ // 18 //
divyadehaḥ sutejasvī divyagandhastvarogavān //
sampūrṇahṛdaye śūnye tvārambhe yogavān bhavet // 19 //

Tr. Attaining the *ārambha* state, a *yogī* develops a lustrous physique, profound insight, complete wellness, sweet fragrance, contentment in heart, while enjoying void. He has the *brahmarandhra* pierced, *nāda* emanating from *sūrya* and he hears a divine unstruck tinkling sound. 18-19.

Note: This verse has a similarity with the verse in HP (iv. 70). However, instead of the word '*brahmarandhre*', HP gives '*brahmagranther*', which seems to be appropriate in the light of the mention of *viṣṇugranthi* and *rudragranthi* in the verses 21 and 24 respectively. 18.

[7]द्वितीयायां घटीकृत्य वायुर्भवति मध्यगः ॥
दृढासनो[8] भवेद् योगी कामदेवसमस्तदा[9] ॥ 20 ॥
विष्णुग्रन्थेस्तथा[10] भेदः परमानन्दसूचकः ॥
अतिशून्ये विमर्दश्च भेरीशब्दस्तथा भवेत्[11] ॥ 21 ॥

dvitīyāyāṃ ghaṭīkṛtya vāyurbhavati madhyagaḥ //
dṛdhāsano bhavedyogī kāmadevasamastadā // 20 //
viṣṇugranthestathā bhedaḥ paramānandasūcakaḥ //
atiśūnye vimardaśca bherīśabdastathā bhavet // 21 //

Tr. In the second state of *ghaṭa*, the *vāyu* (*prāṇa*) passes through the middle path (*suṣumnā*), stability in *āsana* is gained and

---

1. ब्रह्मरन्ध्रैर-t1. 2. आनन्दः-N,n1,J. 3. विचित्रक्वणको-P,T,t1. 4. धृतिः-J. 5. दिव्यगंधात्तवेगवान् -N,n1,J. 6. सम्पूर्णहृदयं-T,t1. 7. अथ घटावस्था–P. 8. दृढासने–P. 9. कामदेवसमस्तथा-P; ज्ञानं देवसमस्तदा-N,n1,n2,J. 10. तदा–P,T. 11. भेरी सदृशस्तदा भवेत्-N,J, भेरीसदृक् सदा -J.

the *yogī* becomes like a cupid. Moreover, the *viṣṇu-granthi* is pierced through, various sounds like that of kettle drum etc. are heard in the void (*atiśūnya*), bringing in Absolute Bliss. 20-21.

[1]तृतीयायां ततो नित्यं[2] आविष्कारो[3] मर्द्दलध्वनिः[4] ॥
महाशून्यं ततो याति सर्वसिद्धिसमाश्रयः ॥ 22 ॥
चिदानन्दं ततो जित्वा[5] परमानन्दसम्भवः ॥
दोषदुःखजरामृत्यु[6]क्षुधा[7]निद्राविवर्जितः ॥ 23 ॥

tṛtīyāyāṃ tato nityaṃ āviṣkāro marddaladhvaniḥ //
mahāśūnyaṃ tato yāti sarvasiddhisamāśrayaḥ // 22 //
cidānandaṃ tato jitvā parmānandasambhavaḥ //
doṣaduḥkhajarāmṛtyukṣudhānidrāvivarjitaḥ // 23 //

Tr. In the third state, one hears the sound of kettle drum, (*prāṇa*) reaches the *mahāśūnya* (center of the eyebrows), which results in attainment of all the *siddhis* (supernatural powers). The *yogī* achieves mental happiness, which springs from Absolute Bliss and becomes free from all disorders, sufferings, old age, (premature) death, hunger and thirst. 22-23.

[8]रुद्रग्रन्थिं ततो भित्वा शर्वपीठगतोऽनिलः[9] ॥
निष्पत्तौ वैणवः शब्दः क्वणद्वीणाक्वणो[10] भवेत् ॥ 24 ॥
इत्यारम्भादियोगावस्थानिरूपणम् ।[11]

rudragranthiṃ tato bhitvā śarvapīṭhagato'nilaḥ //
niṣpattau vaiṇavaḥ śabdaḥ kvaṇadvīṇākvaṇo bhavet // 24 //
ityārambhādiyogāvasthānirūpaṇam //

Tr. When the *anila* (*prāṇa*) courses to the *śarvapīṭha* after piercing through the *rudragranthi*, one attains the state of *niṣpatti* in which he hears the notes of finely tuned *vīṇā*. 24.

---

1. अथ परिचयावस्था–P. 2. भित्वा-P,T. 3. विष्करो –t1. 4. नित्यं विश्रामो मर्द्दलध्वनेः-N,J. 5. भित्वा-n3. 6. मृत्युः-P. 7. क्रोध N,n1,n3,J. 8. अथ निष्पत्यवस्था–P. 9. सर्व पीडाविवर्जितः-J,N,T. 10. क्वणाणि तत्क्षणं–J,N,n3, क्वणन्नीतः क्षणं–T,t1. 11. इत्यारम्भादियोगं च-स्थाननिरूपणं–J,N,n1, इत्यारम्भादियोगं च चक्रस्थाननिरूपणम् -n3.

Here ends the description of the yogic states like *ārambha* etc.

Note: The verse iv.24 seems to have been obviously taken from HP (iv-76) where the reading is *śarvapīṭha* instead of *sarvapīṭha*, which is appropriate and hence it is adopted here.

The different developmental stages in *yoga* have been stated to characterize listening of the internally produced sound from grosser to subtler levels.

AR (xxvii.4807-4812) while quoting another *Tantra* text describes four stages (*avasthās*) of *yoga*, which are: *dhvasti, prāpti, saṃvit*, and *prasāda*, which are apperantly quite different from the *avasthās* commonly available in *haṭhayogic* texts. In the stage of *dhvasti*, the results of both good and bad *karma* are attenuated, and the *cetas* (mind) becomes disinterested in the objects. In the *prāpti* stage, all the desires related to perceptible and spiritual world and also those of greed and infatuation are restrained. In the stage of *saṃvit*, the *yogī* knows all the events of the past and future. In the stage of *prāsāda*, the *manas*, five *vāyus*, senses including their objects become pacified. 18-24.

दृष्टिः स्थिरा[1] यस्य विनैव लक्ष्यात्[2]
वायुः स्थिरो यस्य विना प्रयत्नात् ॥
चित्तं स्थिरं यस्य विनावलम्बात्[3]
स एव योगी स गुरुः स सेव्यः ॥ 25 ॥

dṛṣṭiḥ sthirā yasya vinaiva lakṣyāt
vāyuḥ sthiro yasya vinā prayatnāt //
cittaṃ sthiraṃ yasya vināvalambāt
sa eva yogī sa guruḥ sa sevyaḥ // 25 //

Tr. A *yogī* is considered a *guru*, whose gaze is fixed without an object, *vāyu* is steady without effort and the mind is stable without an object of concentration. Such a *yogī* should be accepted as a *guru*. 25.

---

1. धृष्टस्थिरो-T,t1, दृष्टिः स्थिरो –P. 2. लक्ष्या-N,n1,J, लक्ष्ये –n3. 3. विनावलंबनात् -P,t1.

तत्वं बीजं हठं क्षेत्रमौदासीन्यं जलं त्रिभिः ॥
उन्मनी कल्पलतिका सद्य एव फलिष्यति ॥ 26 ॥
tattvaṃ bījaṃ haṭhaṃ kṣetramaudāsīnyaṃ jalaṃ tribhiḥ //
unmanī kalpalatikā sadya eva phaliṣyati // 26 //

Tr. *Tatva* (Self) is the seed, *haṭha* is the soil and indifference is water. This triad facilitates quick growth of the creeper *unmanī*. 26.

वेदशास्त्रपुराणानि सामान्यगणिका इव ॥
एकैव शाम्भवी मुद्रा गुप्ता कुलवधूरिव[1] ॥ 27 ॥
vedaśāstrapurāṇāni sāmānyagaṇikā iva //
ekaiva śambhavī mudrā guptā kulavadhūriva // 27 //

Tr. The *Vedas,* the *śāstras* and the *Purāṇas* are like public women. *Śāmbhavī mudrā* alone is like a noble woman, not exposed to anyone. 27.

एकं सृष्टिमयं बीजमेका मुद्रा[2] च खेचरी ॥
एको देवो निरालम्बः एकावस्था मनोन्मनी ॥ 28 ॥
ekaṃ sṛṣṭimayaṃ bījamekā mudrā ca khecarī //
eko devo nirālambaḥ ekāvasthā manonmanī // 28 //

Tr. There is only one all-pervading *bīja* of the creation (*OM*), there is only one *mudrā* called *khecarī,* there is only one deity—*nirālamba* (*Brahma*) and only one state — *unmanī* (*samādhi*). 28.

मनो यत्र विलीयेत पवनस्तत्र लीयते ॥ **29** ॥
mano yatra vilīyeta pavanstatra līyate // 29 //

Tr. *Pavana* (*prāṇa*) merges therein where mind merges. 29.

पाताले यद्विशति[3] सुषिरं[4] मेरुमूलं[5] तदस्ति[6]
तत्वं चैतद्वदति सुधा[6] तन्मुखं निम्नगानाम् ॥
चन्द्रात्सारं[7] स्रवति[8] वपुषस्तेन मृत्युर्नराणाम्
तदबध्नीयात्सुखरतिमृदु[9]र्नान्यथा कार्यसिद्धिः[10] ॥ 30 ॥

1. सामान्य - धूरिव -अनुपलब्ध-J,n1,n2,n3. 2. एकं सृष्टिसमुद्बीजमेकावस्था-P,T,t1. 3. चद्वितीयं-P; यद्वितीयं-T. 4. सुषिरे–J. 5. ममरुमूले-P,T, मेरुमूले–J,n1,n3,t1. 6. तदस्मिन्-P,T,t1. 7. तच्चैतन्यं प्रवदति सुधीस्-J,N,n1,n2,n3,n4. 7. चंन्द्रासारं-P,T. 8. पिबति-P,T,t1, श्रवति–J. 9. मृत्युर्-P. 10. कार्यसिद्धः-P.

pātāle yadviśati suṣiraṃ merumūlaṃ tadasti
tatvaṃ caitadvadati sudhā tanmukhaṃ nimnagānām //
candrātsāraṃ sravati vapuṣastenamṛtyurnarāṇām
tadbadhnīyātsukharatimṛdurnānyathā kāryasiddhiḥ /30/

Tr. The learned holds that the aperture, which is located at the base of the spine, is the fountain-head of consciousness. A mortal dies because the ambrosia flowing from the moon moves down. By restraining this with the process giving pleasure (*khecarī mudrā)*, one can attain success (in *laya*) and not otherwise. 30.

Note: This verse seems to have been adopted from HP (iii.51) with a variant reading which is rather confusing. The verse in HP runs as follows:

yatprāleyaṃ prahitasuṣiraṃ merumūrdhāntarastham
tasminstatvaṃ pravadati sudhīstanmukhaṃ nimnagānām /
candrāt sāraḥ sravati vapuṣastena mṛtyurnarāṇāṃ
taṃ badhnīyāt sukaraṇamatho nānyathā kāryasiddhiḥ //

The location of *ātmatatva* is stated to be up in the head and not down below according to *śrutis* and other traditional texts. But here the mention of the location of *ātmatatva* at the base of the spine is misleading.

Similarly, the word *sukaraṇa,* which is a synonym of *khecarī,* is appropriate rather than *sukharati*. 30.

[1]ब्रह्माण्डपिण्डाण्डयोः[2] सांगोपासनयोः[3] पिण्डाण्डस्वरूपं दिङ्मात्रं प्रदर्श्यति[4] |

brahmāṇḍapiṇḍāṇḍayoḥ sāṅgopāsanayoḥ piṇḍāṇḍasvarūpaṃ diṅmātraṃ pradarṣyate //

Tr. A little description follows regarding the microcosmic (individual self) and the macrocosmic nature (of creation) alongwith the technique of its worship :

Note: *Piṇḍa-brahmāṇḍa* is the course taken in the upward march of *kuṇḍalinī.* It is also known as *ṣaṭcakra-mārga.*

शरीरं तावदेवं हि षण्णवत्यंगुलात्मकम् ||
विद्यते सर्वजन्तूनां स्वांगुलिभिरिति प्रिये || 31 ||

---

1. वचनम् -P. 2. ब्रह्माण्डपिण्डयोः-n1. 3 . संख्योपासनाय-P,T,t1. 4. प्रदृश्यते–J,N,n1, इह प्रदर्श्यते–T.

śarīraṃ tāvadevaṃ hi ṣaṇṇavatyaṅgulātmakam //
vidyate sarvajantūnāṃ svāṅgulibhiriti priye // 31 //

Tr. O beloved ! The body of all the creatures would measure nintysix digits by one's own fingers. 31.

Note: The measure of the human body is considered here to be of 96 digits. *Aṅguli* is a measure of three-fourth of an inch. Thus, the body measures six feet. 31.

देहे द्वात्रिंशदस्थीनि शस्तं[1] स्यात्पार्श्वयोर्द्वयोः ॥
द्वासप्तति[2]सहस्राणि नाड्यश्चरति मारुतः ॥ 32 ॥
dehe dvātriṃśadasthīni śastaṃ syātpārśvayordvayoḥ //
dvāsaptatisahasrāṇi nāḍyaśacarati mārutaḥ // 32 //

Tr. There are thirtytwo bones on both the sides (in the back). There are seventytwo thousand *nāḍīs* through which the *māruta* (*prāṇa*) courses. 32.

Note: Instead of the word *śasta*, VS (ii.6) gives the reading *vaṃśasya* (of the bamboo i.e. spine), which is more appropriate. 32.

मूलाधारे स्थितं[3] चक्रं कुक्कुटाण्डमिव स्थितम् ॥
नाडीचक्रमिति प्रोक्तं तस्मान्नाड्यः समागताः ॥ 33 ॥
mūlādhāre sthitaṃ cakraṃ kukkuṭāṇḍamiva sthitaṃ //
nāḍīcakramiti proktaṃ tasmānnāḍyaḥ samāgatāḥ // 33 //

Tr. The *cakra*, resembling an egg of a hen, is located at the *mūlādhāra*, which is called *nāḍīcakra*, wherefrom the *nāḍīs* originate. 33.

नाडीनामपि सर्वासां मुख्यास्तत्र चतुर्दश ॥
सुषुम्णा पिंगला चैव सरस्वती तथा कुहुः[4] ॥ 34 ॥
यशस्विनी वारुणी[5] च गान्धारी शंखिनी[6] तथा ॥
पूषा विश्वोदरी जिह्वा अलम्बुषा च हंसिनी[7] ॥
इडा नाडी च सर्वासां मुख्याश्चैताश्चतुर्दश ॥ 35 ॥
nāḍīnāmapi sarvāsāṃ mukhyāstatra caturdaśa //
suṣumṇā piṅgalā caiva sarasvatī tathā kuhuḥ // 34 //

---

1. शतं -n1, शतं (शस्तं)-P, स्थानशतं–T, द्वात्रिंशतस्थाने शतं –t1. 2. द्विसप्तति–P. 3. स्थिरं-N,n3,J. 4. कुहूः-J,P,n1. 5. दारुणी-N,n3,J; तारुणी-T,t1. 6. शंकिनी-P,T,t1. 7. सिंहिनी-N,n1,n3, J.

yaśasvinī vāruṇī ca gāndhārī śaṅkhinī tathā //
pūṣā viśvodarī jihvā alambuṣā ca haṃsinī //
iḍā nāḍī ca sarvāsāṃ mukhyāścaitāścaturdaśa // 35 //

Tr. Among all the *nāḍīs,* fourteen are prominent, which are—*Suṣumṇā, piṅgalā, sarasvatī, kuhu, yaśasvinī, vāruṇī, gāndhārī, śaṅkhinī, pūṣā, viśvodarī, jihvā, alambuṣā, haṃsinī* and *iḍā.* These fourteen are the most significant. 34-35.

तासां मुख्यतमास्तिस्रः तिसृष्वेकोत्तमा[1] स्थिता ॥
इडायां पिंगलायां च सोमसूर्यौ प्रतिष्ठितौ ॥ 36 ॥
tāsāṃ mukhyatamāstisraḥ tisṛṣvekottamā sthitā //
iḍāyāṃ piṅgalāyāṃ ca somasūryau pratiṣṭhitau // 36 //

Tr. Among these three *nāḍīs* are of great significance, out of which one is the most important. *Soma* and *sūyra* are situated in *iḍā* and *piṅgalā* (respectively). 36.

तामसो राजसश्चैव सव्यदक्षिणसंस्थितौ[2] ॥
इडा निशाकरी ज्ञेया[3] पिंगला[4] सूर्यरूपिणी[5] ॥ 37 ॥
tāmaso rājasaścaiva savyadakṣiṇasaṃsthitau //
iḍā niśākarī jñeyā piṅgalā sūryarūpiṇī // 37 //

Tr. *Nāḍīs* located at the left and right are known as *tāmasa* and *rājasa* respectively. *Iḍā* is of the nature of moon and *piṅgalā* is of the nature of sun. 37.

वीणादण्डमयो मेरुरस्थीनि[6] कुलपर्वताः ॥
इडा भागीरथी प्रोक्ता पिंगला यमुना नदी[7] ॥ 38 ॥
सरस्वती सुषुम्नोक्ता नाड्योऽन्या निम्नगाः स्मृताः ॥
द्वीपाः स्युर्धातवस्[8]सप्त स्वेदलालादयोर्मयः[9] ॥ 39 ॥
vīṇādaṇḍamayo merurasthīni kulaparvatāḥ //
iḍā bhāgīrathī proktā piṅgalā yamunā nadī // 38 //
sarasvatī suṣumnoktā nāḍyo'nyā nimnagāḥ smṛtāḥ //
dvīpāḥ syurdhātavassapta svedalālādayormayaḥ // 39 //

---

1. तिसृष्वेकतमा-N,n1,n2,n3,n4,J. 2. सव्यदक्षिणसंज्ञकौ–N,n2n3,J,P,T, सम्यग्दक्षिसञ्ज्ञकौ –t1. 3. ज्ञेयौ–P. 4. सुषुम्ना-P,T,J. 5. सुखरूपिणी-P,T, इडा निशाकरी ज्ञेयः सुषुम्नासुखरूपिणी–t1. 6. दारुरस्थिनी-P,T,t1. 7. द्वे प्रकीर्त्तिते–P,T,t1, गंगा च पिंगला नाडी यमुनेडा प्रकीर्त्तिताः–N,J. 8. र्द्धानवस्-J. 9. स्वेदलाला द्वयोर्द्वयोः -P,T,t1.

Tr. Bones of the spine resemble a *vīṇā*, wherein the *kulaparvatas* (mountains) are located. The *piṅgalā nāḍī* is *gaṅgā*, while *iḍā* is *yamunā* and *suṣumnā* is *sarasvatī*. Other (*nāḍīs*) flow downwards. The seven *dhātus* (body constituents) are *dvīpas* (islands) replete with saliva, sweat etc. 38-39.

मूले तिष्ठति कालाग्निः[1] कपाले चन्द्रमण्डलम् ॥
नक्षत्राण्यपराण्याहुरेवं योज्यं तु धीमता ॥ 40 ॥
mūle tiṣṭhati kālāgniḥ kapāle candramaṇḍalam //
nakṣatrāṇyaparāṇyāhurevaṃ yojyaṃ tu dhīmatā // 40 //

Tr. *Kālāgni* (fire) is located at the base (*mūlādhāra*), while *candra* (moon) is located in the forehead. The wise should similarly locate other stars also. 40.

ग्रन्थविस्तारभीत्या तु नास्माभिरिह लिख्यते ॥
granthavistārabhītyā tu nāsmābhiriha likhyate //

Tr. All the details are not put forth considering that it would inflate the volume of the book.

श्रुत्यागमपुराणाद्यैः पिण्डब्रह्माण्डनिर्णयः ॥[2]
ज्ञातव्यः[3] सर्वयत्नेन मोक्षसाम्राज्यमिच्छता[4] ॥ 41 ॥

इति पिण्डाण्डयोः किञ्चित् साम्यदर्शनम् ॥

śrutyāgamapurāṇādyaiḥ piṇḍabrahmāṇḍanirṇayaḥ //
jñātavyaḥ sarvayatnena mokṣasāmrājyamicchatā // 41 //

iti piṇḍāṇḍayoḥ kiñcit sāmyadarśanam //

Tr. The account of microcosmic (individual body) and macrocosmic nature should be known from the *śrutis*, *āgamas* and *purāṇas* etc., which one should learn to reign over the kingdom of emancipation. 41.

Here ends the terse but accurate account of mirocosmic *(piṇḍa)* and macrocosmic *(brahmāṇḍa)* body.

---

1. ' —वस्ति मध्ये तु (बांधवः) वाडवः । वैद्युताग्निः सुषुम्नायां पार्थिवो नाभिमण्डले । हृदि तिष्ठति कालाग्निः'- P,T,t1. 2. द्रष्टव्यम् परिशिष्टम् 1. 3. ज्ञेयं –n3. 4. इच्छुना-P.

[1]अथ पञ्चीकरणम्[2] —
शब्दाद् व्योम स्पर्शतत्वेन[3] वायुस्ताभ्यां[4] रूपाद् वह्निरेतैरसाच्च ॥
अम्भांस्येभिर्गन्धतो भूधराद्या भूताः पञ्च स्युर्गुणानुक्रमेण ॥ 42 ॥
***atha pañcīkaraṇam* —**
śabdād vyoma sparśatatvena vāyus-
tābhyāṃ rūpād vahniretairasācca //
ambhāṃsyebhirgandhato bhūdharādyā
bhūtāḥ pañca syurguṇānukrameṇa // 42 //

Tr. From *śabda* emanated *ākāśa* (space), from *sparśa* (touch) emanated *vāyu*, from these two and *rūpa* (form) emanated *vahni* (fire), from these and *rasa* (taste) emanated *ambhas* (water) and from these and *gandha* (smell) emanated *bhū* (earth). Thus the five *bhūtas* evolved from these *guṇas* in their order. 42.

Note: This process is clearly mentioned in HP (10 chapters i.18-25, published by Lonavla Yoga Institue, India), which is as follows:

"*Ākāśa* (ether) is the foremost of the immutable evolutes, characterised by *śabda*. *Vāyu*, which is emanated from *ākāśa*, is fickle and has the quality of touch. *Tejas*, which is the evolute of both *ākāśa* and *vāyu*, is qualified by form. *Āpa* (water), which is originated from *ākāśa*, *vāyu* and *agni*, is characterized by taste. *Pṛthvī*, which has been evolved from *ākāśa*, *vāyu*, *tejas* and *āpa*, has the quality of smell".

This is the evolution of the five *mahābhūtas* according to their *guṇas* (qualities). 42.

कर्पूरमनले[5] यद्वत् सैन्धवं सलिले यथा ॥[6]
तथा सन्धीयमानं हि मनस्तत्रैव लीयते ॥ 43 ॥
karpūramanale yadvat saindhavaṃ salile yathā //

1. वचनम् - अथ पिण्डीकरणम् प्रक्रिया दिङ्मात्रं प्रदर्श्यते-P,T,t1. 2. वचनम्-P. 3. शब्दाद्व्योमरस स्पर्शस्तेन-P,T, n1. 4. 'रूपाद इत्यादि' ... 'गुणानुक्रमेण' अनुपलब्ध-P,T. 5. कर्पूरं सलिले –N,n1,n3,n4,J, कर्पूरकमनले -P. 6. पंक्तिः अनुपलब्धा-T.

tathā sandhīyamānaṃ hi manastatraiva līyate // 43 //

Tr. Just as camphor merges in fire and salt dissolves in water, similarly, mind focused on it (*Brahma*), gets merged with it . 43.

ज्ञेयवस्तुपरित्यागाद्विलयं[1] याति मानसः[2] ||
मानसे विलयं याते कैवल्यमुपजायते || 44 ||[3]
jñeyavastuparityāgādvilayaṃ yāti mānasaḥ //
mānase vilayaṃ yāte kaivalyamupajāyate // 44 //

Tr. On giving up the objects of perception, mind merges (in the Absolute). On dissolution of mind, *kaivalya* alone prevails. 44.

खमध्ये कुरु चात्मानमात्ममध्ये च खं कुरु ||
सर्वं च खमयं कृत्वा न किञ्चिदपि चिन्तयेत्[4] || 45 ||
khamadhye kuru cātmānamātmamadhye ca khaṃ kuru //
sarvaṃ ca khamayaṃ kṛtvā na kiñcidapi cintayet // 45 //

Tr. Merge the *Ātmā* into void and void into *Ātmā*. Perceive the void everywhere and do not think of anything else. 45.

अन्तः पूर्णो बहिः पूर्णः पूर्णकुम्भ इवाम्भसि ||[5]
अन्तः शून्यं बहिः शून्यं शून्यकुम्भ इवाम्बरे || 46 ||
antaḥ pūrṇo bahiḥ pūrṇaḥ pūrṇakumbha ivāmbhasi //
antaḥ śūnyaṃ bahiḥ śūnyaṃ śūnyakumbha ivāmbare // 46 //

Tr. Just as a filled pitcher drowned in water has the water in and out, similarly perceive the void in and out like an empty pitcher in the space. 46.

स्वगतेनैव कालिम्ना दर्पणं मलिनं यथा[6] ||
अज्ञानेनावृतं ज्ञानं तेन मुह्यन्ति जन्तवः ||[7]
एक एव हि भूतात्मा भूते भूते व्यवस्थितः || 47 ||
svagatenaiva kālimnā darpaṇaṃ malinaṃ yathā //
ajñānenāvṛtaṃ jñānaṃ tena muhyanti jantavaḥ //
eka eva hi bhūtātmā bhūte bhūte vyavasthitaḥ // 47 //

---

1. ज्ञेयवस्तुपरित्यागः विलयं–P. 2.मानसं–J,P,n4. 3.उत्तरार्धः अनुपलब्धः-P,T,t1.
4.'चिन्तयेत्' अनुपलब्धः-T. 5.पंक्तिः अनुपलब्धा -P,T,t1. 6. तथा–N,J.
7. अनुपलब्धपंक्तिः-N,n1,n4,J.

Tr. Just as the reflection (mirror) appears tarnished due to the face having been coloured, similarly, ignorance conceals wisdom due to which people are illusioned. The same cosmic Self is located in every creature. 47.

एकधा बहुधा चैव दृश्यते[1] जलचन्द्रवत् ॥
मायायुक्तस्तथा जीवो मायाहीनसदा शिवः[2] ॥ 48 ॥
ekadhā bahudhā caiva dṛśyate jalacandravat //
māyāyuktastathā jīvo māyāhīnas-sadāśivaḥ // 48 //

Tr. As the reflection of the moon in water is perceived as one as well as many, so also, the *jīva* (embodied self) being attached to attributes (*māyā*= illusion) is *jīva* and without attributes it is *Sadāśiva*. 48.

बन्ध[3]मोक्षोपदेशादिव्यवहारोऽपि मायया ॥
मायाच्छेदः[4] प्रकर्तव्यः सुदृढं ज्ञानयोगतः[5] ॥ 49 ॥
bandhamokṣopadeśādivyavahāro'pi māyayā //
māyācchedaḥ prakartavyaḥ sudṛḍhaṃ jñānayogataḥ // 49 //

Tr. Even the attributes like bondage and liberation, as conventionally used, are due to *māyā* (ignorance). *Māyā* should be severed by firm resolution of *jñāna-yoga*. 49.

अत्र सूतसंहितायाम्[6] —
एतदात्ममिदं[7] सर्वं नेह नानास्ति किञ्चन[8] ॥
अद्वैतमेव शास्त्रार्थः शम्भोः पादं स्पृशाम्यहम् ॥ 50 ॥
atra sūtasaṃhitāyām —
etadātmamidaṃ sarvaṃ neha nānāsti kiñcana //
advaitameva śāstrārthaḥ śambhoḥ pādaṃ spṛśāmyaham /50/
According to *Sūtasaṃhitā*—

Tr. It is all but one *Ātmā*, and there is no multiplicity. The contention of all the scriptures is the one Absolute (*Advaita*). I touch the feet of *Śaṃbhu*. 50.

---

1. दृश्यतेव-J. 2. तथाशिवः-P,T,n4. 3 .बिन्दु-P,T,t1. 4. मायाच्छेद–J,T,n1. 5 .योगमिच्छता-N,n1,n3,n4,J. 6. अत्र सूतसंहिता–P,n4. 7. तत्तदात्ममिदं–P,T,t1. 8 .नेहनानास्तिकं च-N.

विष्णुपुराणे[1] —

कनकमुकुटकर्णिकादिभेदः कनकमभिन्नमपीष्यते यथैकम्[2] ॥

बुधपशुमनुजादिकल्पभिन्नो हरिरखिलाभिरुदीर्यते तथैकम्[3] ॥ 51 ॥

जीवात्मपरमात्मनोरपि भेदोपासनायामपि[4] ॥

***viṣṇupurāṇe* —**

kanakamukuṭakarṇikādibhedaḥ
kanakamabhinnamapīṣyate yathaikam //
budhapaśumanujādikalpabhinno
harirakhilābhirudīryate tathaikam // 51 //

***jīvātmaparamātmanorapi bhedopāsanāyāmapi* //**

According to *Viṣṇupurāṇa*—

Tr. As gold can be found in bracelet, crown, earring etc., similarly, Cosmic Soul, called *hari,* is pervading in planets (lit. Mercury), animals and human beings. 51.

In the same manner, the difference in *jīvātma* and *Paramātmā* persists even in *upāsanā.*

भगवद्गीतायाम्[5] –

उत्तमः पुरुषस्त्वन्यः परमात्मेत्युदाहृतः ॥

यो लोकत्रयमाविश्य बिभर्त्यव्यय ईश्वरः ॥ 52 ॥

तन्मते[6] दिङ्मात्र[7]स्वरूपप्रदर्शननिराकरणम् ॥

***bhagavadgītāyām* —**

uttamaḥ puruṣastvanyaḥ paramātmetyudāhṛtaḥ //
yo lokatrayamāviśya bibhartyavyaya īśvaraḥ // 52 //

***tanmate diṅmātrasvarūpapradarśananirākaraṇam* //**

According to *Bhagavadgītā* —

Tr. The Superior *Puruṣa* is called *Paramātmā.* One, that pervades and sustains the three worlds, that is immutable, is *Īśvara.* 52.

---

1. विष्णुपुराणेऽपि –P,T. 2. यथैकम् -अनुपलब्धः-P,T,t1. 3. तथैकः-P,t1. 4. जीवत्मपरमात्मनोरपि भेदोपासनामपि –N,J. 5. भगवद्गीता–J,N,n4,T. 6. तत्तन्मते-P,T. 7. दिङ्मात्रं –P,T.

This much is enough to repudiate diversities of the views.

भूतैश्च पञ्चभिर्प्राणै[1]श्चतुर्विंशदभि[2]रिन्द्रियैः ॥
चतुर्विंशति तत्वानि सांख्यशास्त्रविदो विदुः ॥ 53 ॥
bhūtaiśca pañcabhirprāṇaiścaturviṃśadbhirindriyaiḥ //
caturviṃśati tatvāni sāṃkhyaśāstravido viduḥ // 53 //

Tr. The twenty-four *tatvas* include five *bhūtas, prāṇas* and *indriyas.*

According to *Sāṃkhya*, the *tatvas* are twenty four. 53.

अहंकारं प्रधानं च माया विद्या च पूरुषः ॥
इति पौराणिकाः प्राहुः त्रिंशत्तत्वानि तैः सह ॥ 54 ॥
ahaṃkāraṃ pradhānaṃ ca māyā vidyā ca pūruṣaḥ //
iti paurāṇikāḥ prāhuḥ triṃśattatvāni taiḥ saha // 54 //

Tr. *Paurāṇikas* consider thirty *tatvas* inclusive of *ahaṃ kāra, māyā, vidyā* and *Puruṣa* etc. 54.

बिन्दुनादौ शक्तिशिवौ शाम्भवीति ततः परम् ॥
षद्त्रिंशत्तत्वमित्युक्तं[3] शैवागमविशारदैः ॥ 55 ॥
bindunādau śaktiśivau śāṃbhavīti tataḥ param //
ṣaṭtriṃśattatvamityuktaṃ śaivāgamaviśāradaiḥ // 55 //

Tr. The experts of *Śaivāgama* have stated thirty six *tatvas*, in which *bindu, nāda, śiva, śakti* and *śāṃbhavī* are included. 55.

Note: The number of *tatvas* differ in different tradition and different texts. The narration of *tatvas* by *Śrīnivāsa* may be considered as optional. 53-55.

उपादानं प्रपञ्चस्य संसक्ताः परमाणवः ॥
पूर्णरूपादयस्तेषां[4] तेभ्यो जाता घटादयः ॥ 56 ॥

---

1. प्राणाश्च-P,T. 2. चतुर्विंशतिरि–P,t1. 3. षड्विंशत्तत्वमित्युक्तं–n1.
4. गुणरूपादयस्तेषां-P.

upādānaṃ prapañcasya saṃsaktāḥ paramāṇavaḥ //
pūrṇarūpādayasteṣāṃ tebhyo jātā ghaṭādayaḥ // 56 //

Tr. The *paramāṇus* (atoms), coming together, are the cause of the *prapañca* (perceptible world). They contain the quality and form, wherefrom *ghaṭa* (pot) etc., take shape. 56.

यत्कार्यं जायते यस्मात्तत्तत्तस्मिन् प्रतिष्ठितम्[1] ॥
मृत्तिकायां घटस्तन्तौ पटस्स्वर्णेऽङ्गुलीयकम् ॥ 57 ॥[2]
इति वैशेषिकाः[3] प्राहुस्तथा नैयायिका अपि[4] ॥
जनार्दनाख्यमिश्राश्च भट्टाः प्राभाकरादयः ॥ 58 ॥

yatkāryaṃ jāyate yasmāttattattasmin pratiṣṭhitam //
mṛttikāyāṃ ghaṭastantau paṭassvarṇe'ṅgulīyakam // 57 //
iti vaiśeṣikāḥ prāhustathā naiyāyikā api //
janārdanākhyamiśrāśca bhaṭṭāḥ prābhākarādayaḥ // 58 //

Tr. The effect is embedded therein wherefrom it has been originated, like a pot is embedded in soil, cloth in fibre and a ring in gold. This is supported both by *Vaiśeṣikas* and *Naiyāyikas*, so also by the followers of *Janārdana Miśras* and *Bhāṭṭa-prābhākara* etc. 57-58.

ईश्वरस्य तु कर्तृत्वं नांगीचक्रुश्च मण्डनाः[5] ॥ 59 ॥
īśvarasya tu kartṛtvaṃ nāṅgīcakruśca maṇḍanāḥ // 59 //

Tr. The followers of *Maṇḍana* do not agree that *Īśvara* is the cause (of the phenomenal creation). 59.

सत्वं रजस्तमश्चेति प्रधानास्त्रिगुणास्त्रयः ॥
तेभ्यो जातमिदं[6] विश्वं सृष्टिस्थित्यन्तहेतवः ॥ 60 ॥
sattvaṃ rajastamaśceti pradhānastriguṇāstrayaḥ //
tebhyo jātamidaṃ viśvaṃ sṛṣṭisthityantahetavaḥ // 60 //

Tr. Primarily, there are three *guṇas*, such as *satva, rajas* and *tamas,* wherefrom this Universe has been evolved and which hold the key to creation, sustenance and dissolution. 60.

---

1. यस्मात्तस्मिन्प्रतितिष्ठति-P. 2. श्लोकः अनुपलब्धः-T. 3. वैशेषिकः-P. 4. अपिच -P. 5. मण्डलाः-P,T. 6. तेभ्यो जायते-P,T,t1.

मायाप्रधानमव्यक्तमविद्याज्ञानमक्षरम्[1] ॥
अव्याकृतं[2] च प्रकृतिस्तम इत्यभिधीयते ॥ 61 ॥
māyāpradhānamavyaktamavidyājñānamakṣaram //
avyākṛtaṃ ca prakṛtistama ityabhidhīyate // 61 //

Tr. *Māyā, pradhāna, avyakta, avidyā, ajñāna, akṣara, avyākṛta, prakṛti* and *tamas* are the synonymous. 61.

इति सांख्याश्च भाषन्ते तेषां दूषणमुच्यते ॥
चैतन्यं परमाणूनां प्रधानस्यापि नेष्यते ॥ 62 ॥
iti sāṃkhyāśca bhāṣante teṣāṃ dūṣaṇamucyate //
caitanyaṃ paramāṇūnāṃ pradhānasyāpi neṣyate // 62 //

Tr. This (view) is held by the *Sāṃkhyas*, drawback of which is as follows. It is not acceptable that *paramāṇu* (atoms) or even *pradhāna* (the Primal) should have Consciousness (*caitanya*). 62.

ज्ञानशक्तिक्रियाशक्त्या[3] दृश्यते चेतनाश्रयः[4] ॥
तस्मादात्मन[5] आकाशः सम्भूत इति विश्रुतः[6] ॥ 63 ॥
jṇānaśaktikriyāśaktyā dṛśyate cetanāśrayaḥ //
tasmādātmana ākāśaḥ sambhūta iti viśrutaḥ // 63 //

Tr. Consciousness can be perceived through *jñānaśakti* and *kriyāśakti.* It is held in the *śruti* that *ākāśa* is originated from *Ātmā*. 63.

Note: ***Kriyāśakti***—There are three forms of occult power, namely, *manojavitva* (doing any act at any time), *kāmarūpitva* (assuming any form at will), and *vikaraṇadharmitva* (infinite mental power to consume and transmit).

Jñānaśakti—The power of knowledge, which according to *Vīra-śaivas*, is associated with *guruliṅga*, symbolizing the perspective modification of the supreme being. 63.

---

1. ज्ञानमक्षरी –t1. 2. अव्याकृतिं–P,T,t1. 3. ज्ञानक्रिया क्रियाशक्त्या -P,T,t1, ज्ञानशक्तिः क्रियाशक्त्या -n1. 4. चेतनाश्रये –P,T,t1, चेतनाश्रया–n1. 5. तस्मादात्मनश्चा-N. 6. विश्रुतिः-J,N,n1,n3.

शैवाः पाशुपता महाव्रतधराः कालामुखा जंगमाः
शाक्ताः कौल[1]कुलार्चना विधिरताश्चान्येऽपि वा[2] वादिनः ||[3]
एते कृत्रिमतन्त्रतत्वनिरता[4]स्तत्तत्वतो वञ्चितास्
तस्मात्सिद्धिपदं स्वभावनिरतं धीरः सदा[5] संश्रयेत् || 64 ||

śaivāḥ pāśupatā mahāvratadharāḥ kālāmukhā jaṅgamāḥ
śāktāḥ kaulakulārcanā vidhiratāścānye'pi vā vādinaḥ //
ete kṛtrimatantratatvaniratāstattatvato vaṇcitās
tasmāt siddhipadaṃ svabhāvaniratam dhīraḥ sadā saṃśrayet // 64 //

Tr. The *Śaivas, Pāśupatas, Mahāvratadharas, Kālāmukhas, Jaṅgamas, Śāktas, Kaulakulārcanas, Vidhiratas* and such other learned are engaged in futile courses of artificial sciences and hence are far away from the Truth (*tatva*). Therefore, the wise should always take recourse to *siddhipada* (*yoga*), which is very much innate. 64.

Note: *Śaiva*— Followers of *Śaivism*, the most influential cult in south India. *Śaivite* scriptures are collectively referred to as the *Śaivāgama. Śaivite* cults are generally more ascetic. There are orthodox forms as well as perverted forms of *Śaivite* sects. They radically differ from each other. The veneration of *liṅga* is an integral part of most *Śaivite* sects.

Pāśupata—One of the earlier forms of *Śaiva* system. The ultimate cause is believed to be *Śiva,* who is omniscient, omnipresent and almighty. The world, or individual (*paśu*) fails to recognize him owing to *pāśa* or fetters. All the problems and conditions of worldly existence can be solved by a proper comprehension of the five main tenets of this system—*kārya, kāraṇa, yoga, vidhi* and *duḥkhānta*.

---

1. काल -P,N,n1. 2. यो -P. 3. पंक्तिः अनुपलब्धाः-T,t1. 4. तन्त्रनिरतास् -P,T, कृत्रिमतन्त्रनित्यनिरतास् -t1. 5. धीरस्य वा-P.

Mahāvratadhara—Followers of the (persons participating in) functions on the second day in a *satra* ritual in which certain features of primitive collective life can be clearly observed. A *mahāvrata* cup of *soma* is offered and *mahāvratasāman* is chanted, while the priests sway in tune with the rhythmic chanting during the ritual. An *Ārya* and a *Śūdra* should engage themselves in a mock fight while a harlot and a *brahmacārī* should abuse each other. Sexual intercourse between a selected man and woman should take place in a screened shed after which there is drum-beating, singing and dancing.

Mahāvratadhara is a designation for the *Kāpālikas.*

Kālamukha—An extremist *Śaiva* sect mentioned by *Rāmānuja, Keśava Kaśmirī, Haribhadra* and others. This sect existed together with *Pāśupata* order between 11th and 13th centuries in South India at Kāñcī, Tiruvariyur, Melpadi, Kodambalur and other places. *Kālamukhas* existed in two big divisions known as *Śakti-pariṣad* and *Siṃha-pariṣad*, each of which had its own sub-divisions. They had a special relationship with *Nyāya* school of thought.

Kaulamārga—The last of the seven *tāntric ācāras,* which is so influential that it is often equated with Tantrism itself. It is the exclusive cult of *śakti* as the Female principle with the rituals of five Ms or *pañcamakāras*, the aim being the realization of *sāmarasya* of *Śiva* and *śakti* within the Self. *Śrīvidyā* and her forms are the principal objects of this cult. In some texts, it is regarded as anti-vedic and imported from China. The Tantric texts distinguish two categories of *Kaulamārga*. They also describe in detail the qualification and competence of aspirants, nature of spiritual exercise, physical and mental fitness required in this cult, the *kaula* theory of knowledge, its attitude towards woman, its secrecy, warn against its misuse.

Kulārcanā— Followers of the cult of *śakti* as the female Principle with the rituals of Five Ms or *pañcamakāras,* the aim being the realization of *sāmarasya* (identity) of *Śiva* and *Śakti* within the Self.

Jaṅgama—A *Śaiva* sect mentioned in *Ānandagiri's Śaṅkaravijaya.*

Vidhirata—Those who are engaged in the fourth category of the *Pāśupata* system which means the ways to achieve the end. The important *vidhis* are known as *caryās*, which are again subdivided into *vratas* (vows) and *dvāra* (door). *Vidhi* is also the term for injunction. *Vidhimārga* means the way of injunctions and prohibitions or the path of duties. *Vidhis* are variously classified as *apūrva, Niyama* and *parisaṃkhyā* or into *puruṣārtha* and *kratvartha.* 64.

इति श्रीनिवासयोगीश्वरविरचितायां हठरत्नावल्यां चतुर्थो पदेशः[1]

iti śrīnivāsayogīśvaraviracitāyāṃ haṭharatnāvalyāṃ caturthopadeśaḥ

Here ends the fourth chapter of Haṭharatnāvalī, composed by Śrīnivāsa Yogīśvara

---

1. श्रीमत्तार्किकचूडामणिधरणीशकर्णव्याख्यावेदान्त-परिभाषाद्यनेक-प्रबन्धकरण-जन्यजयलक्ष्मी-विराजमानहठयोग-प्रवर्त्तकाचार्यः तिम्मय-ज्योतिषिकसोमाम्बात्मज-श्रीनिवासभट्टयोगीन्द्रविरचितायां श्रीहठरत्नावल्यां चतुर्थोपदेशः // शुभं भवतु // -T, समाप्तस्सम्पूर्णम् शुभम् -N, सम्पूर्ण ॱ समाप्तः -J.
स्वस्तिश्रीसम्वत् १८९५ श्रीशाकसम्वत्सर १७६० / श्रीनेपालसम्वत् ९५९ / मार्गशिरशुपञ्चमीवृहस्पतिवारे इदं रत्नावलीनामग्रन्थलिखितं सम्पूर्णम् / स्वस्ति श्रीविक्रमाब्दे शरग्रहगजभूसम्मिते मार्गशुक्ले, पञ्चम्यां पूर्णतिथौ गुरुदिनदिवसे विश्वमक्षे च गण्डे / धन्वर्के कुम्भलग्ने शशिमकरगते वाग्मतीपूर्वभागे गोडावर्य्युत्तरेहिः हिमगिरियमगे गण्डकीपश्चिमे च /1/ नेपाले मध्यदेशे नगरभगत्पुरे भैरवीमातृकाग्रे दैवज्ञे लेखनियं हठरत्नावलीधर्ममोक्षार्थसिद्धि //- n1.
समाप्तोऽयं ग्रन्थः / श्रीगुरुपादारबिन्दद्वयं नमः / श्रीगोविन्दार्पणमस्तु / इदं पुस्तकं श्रीश्री...../ / -n3.

Illustrations of Āsanas

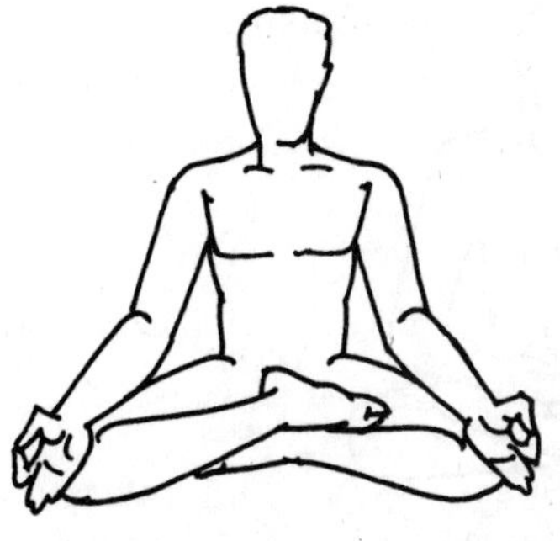
Siddhāsana

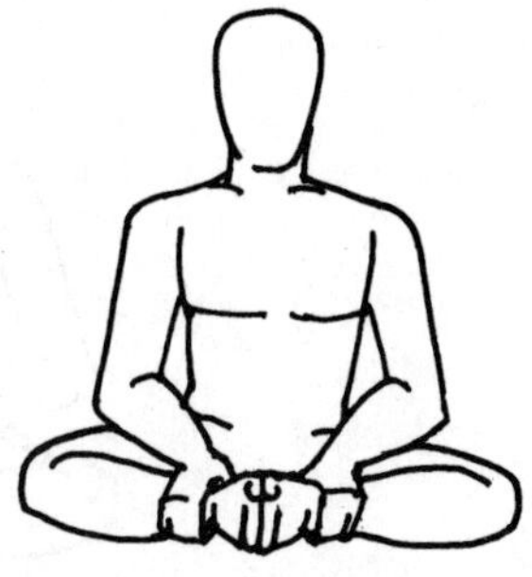
Bhadrāsana

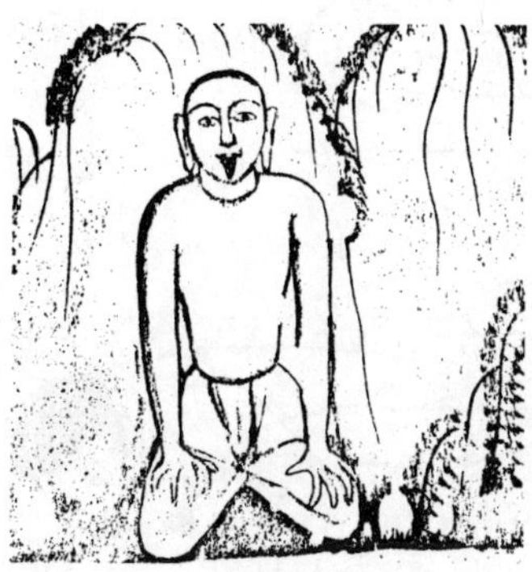
Simhāsana

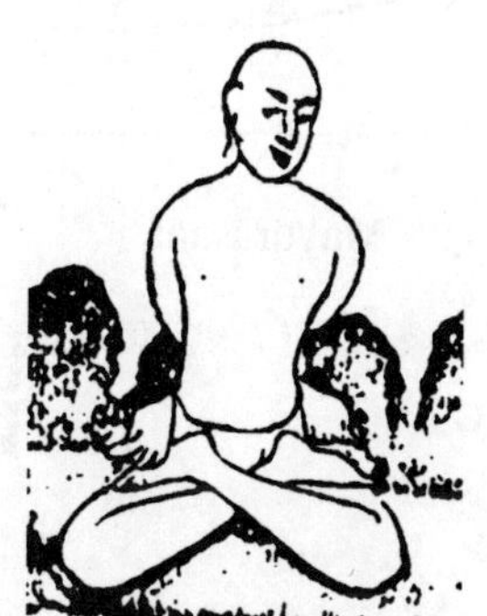
Padmāsana-1

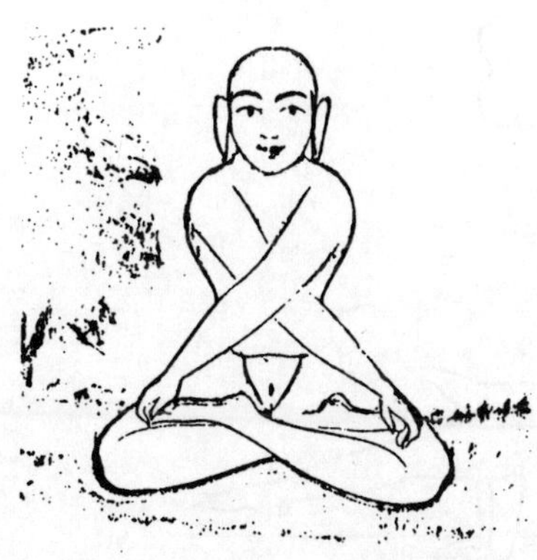
Padmāsana-2

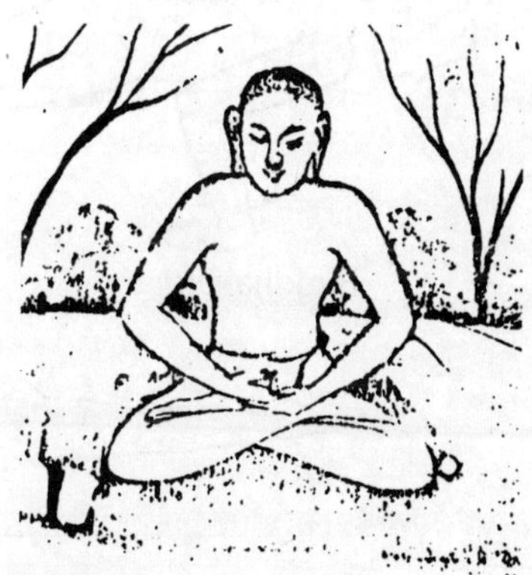
Padmāsana-3

Haṭharatnāvalī

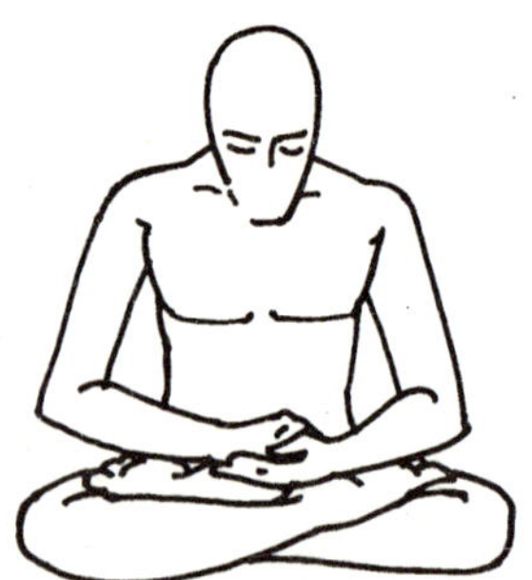

Kara-sampuṭita-padma

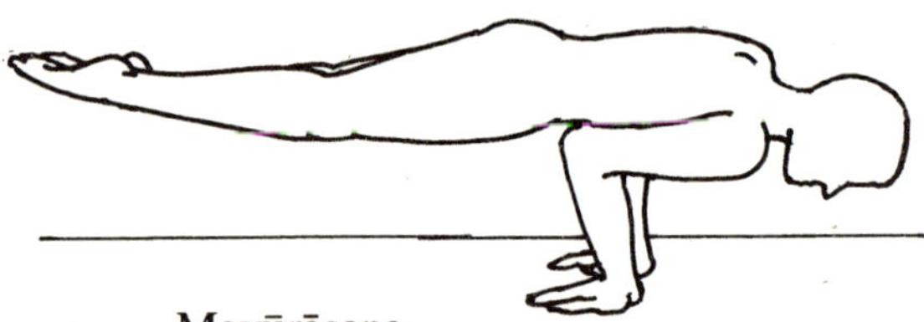

Mayūrāsana

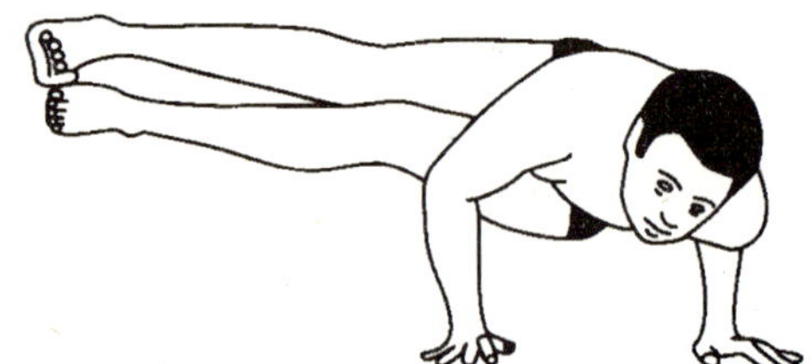

Pārśvamayūra

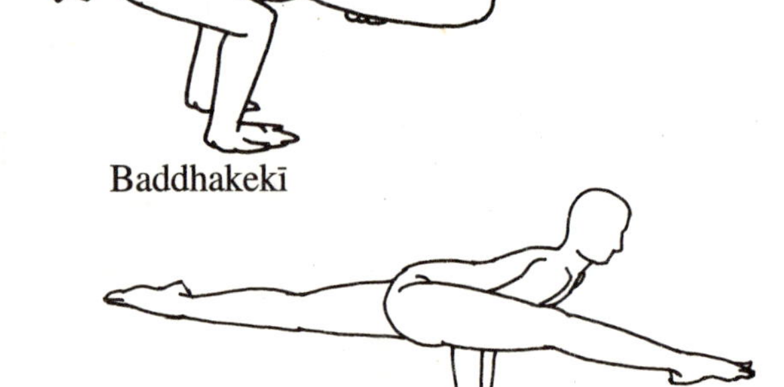

Baddhakekī

Piṇḍamayūra

Illustrations of Āsanas

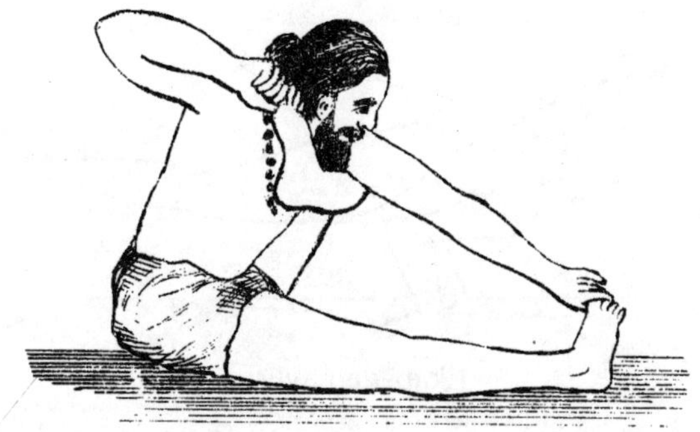

Dhanurāsana

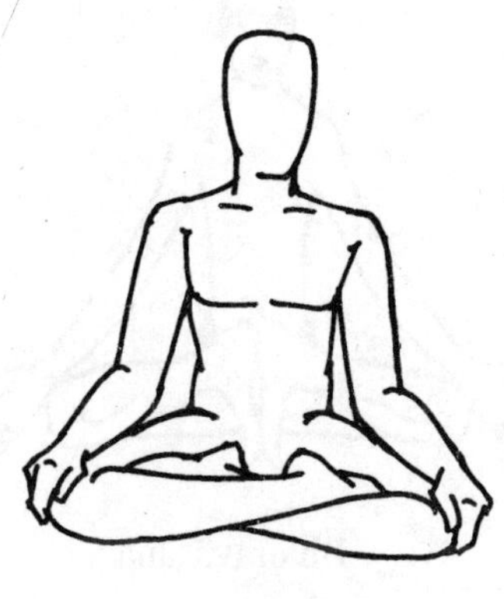

Svastikāsana

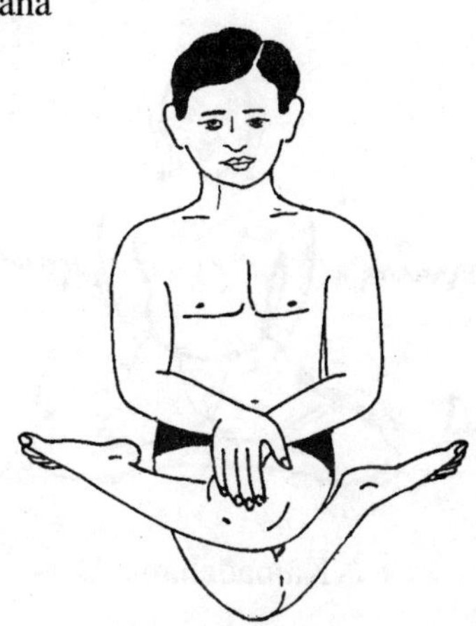

Gomukhāsana

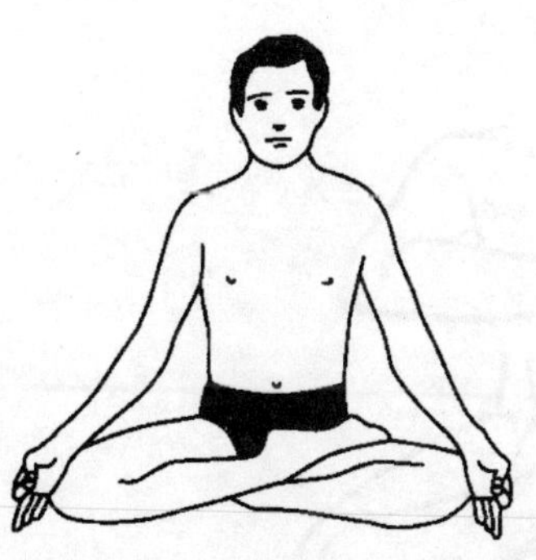

Vīrāsana

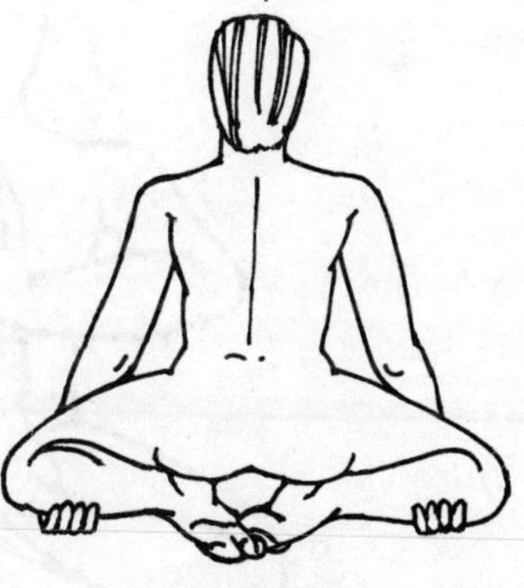

Maṇḍūkāsana

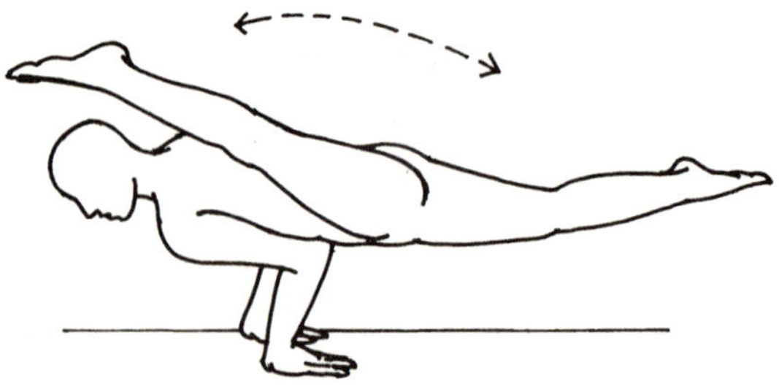

Ekapādamayūra

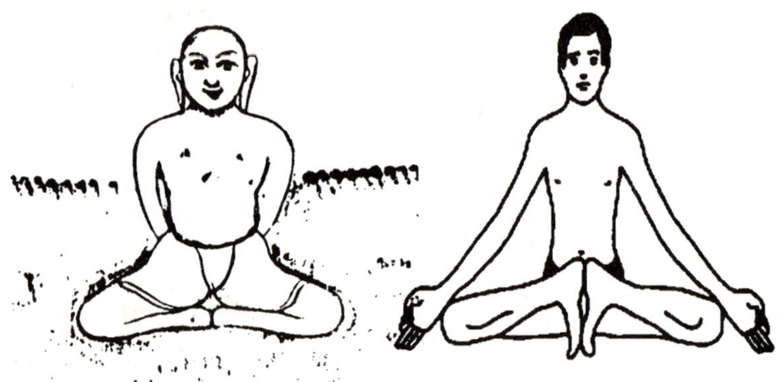

Kāmadahana

Bhairavāsana

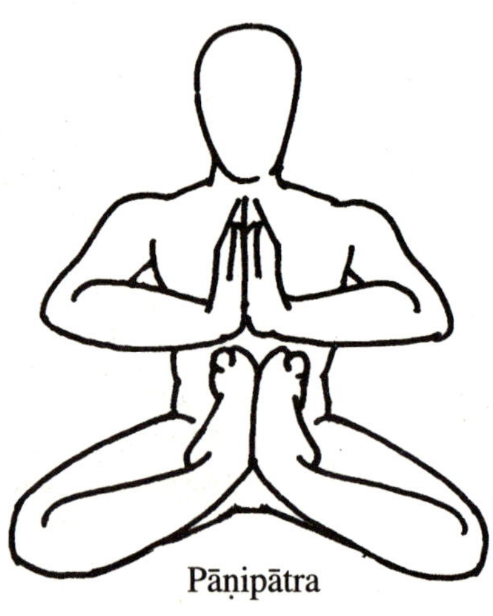

Pāṇipātra

Illustrations of Āsanas

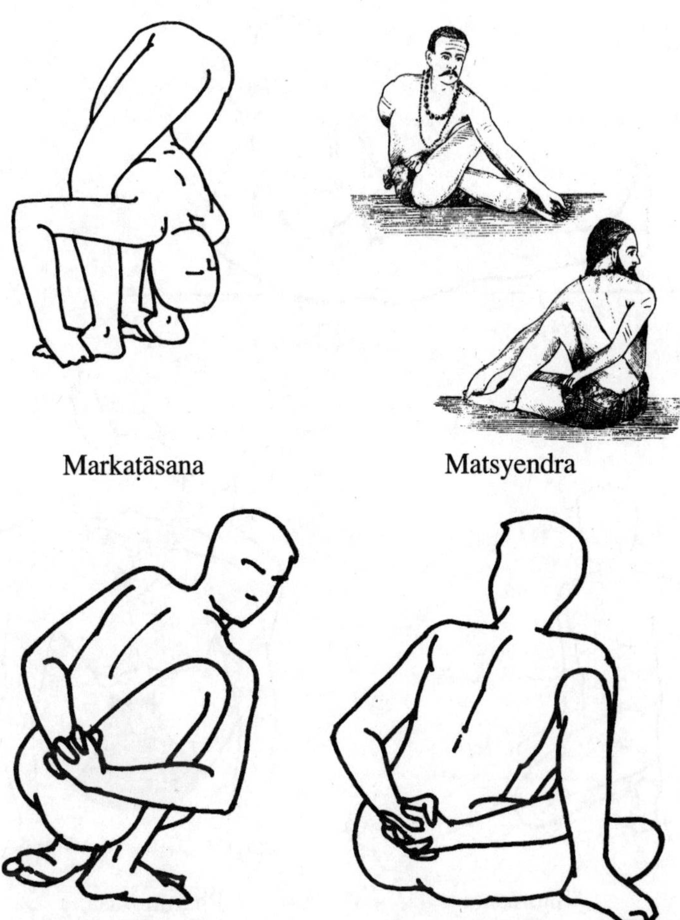

Markaṭāsana

Matsyendra

Pārśvamatsyendra

Baddhamatsyendra

Nirālaṃbana

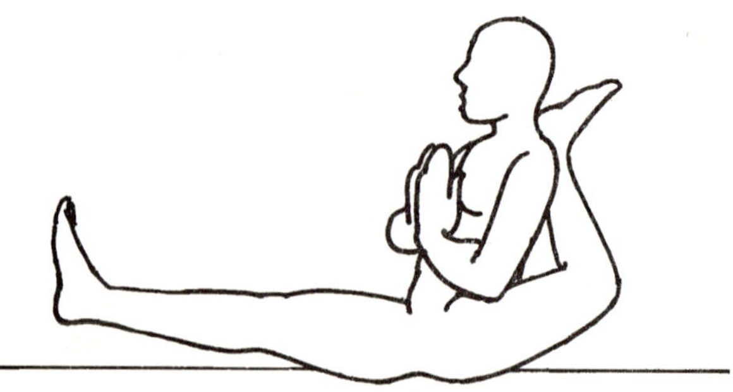

Ekapādāsana

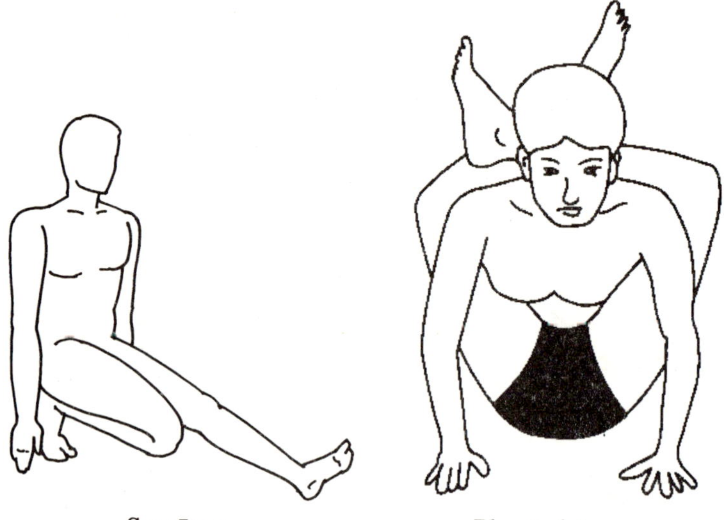

Saurāsana

Phaṇīndrāsana

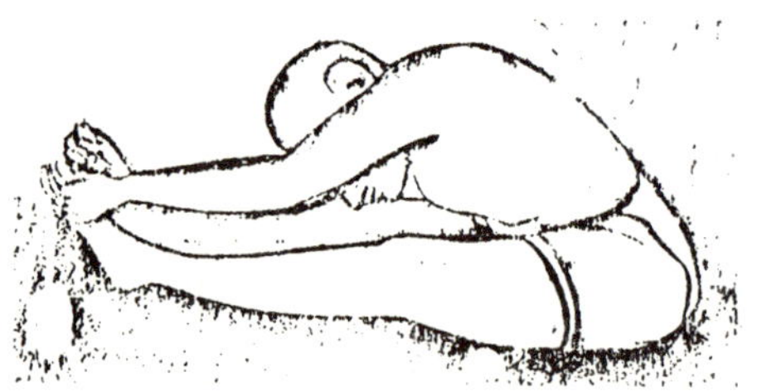

Paścimatāna

Illustrations of Āsanas

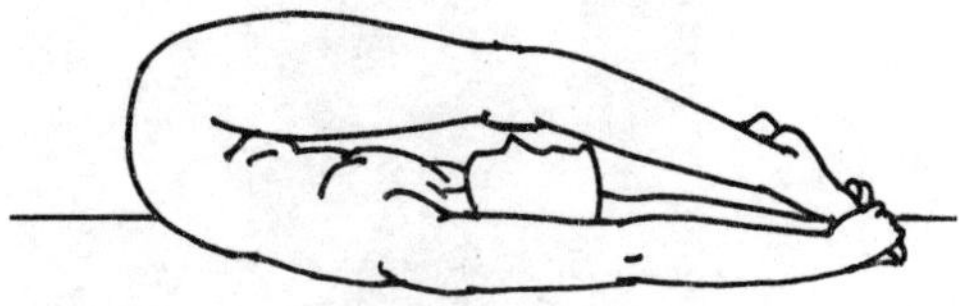

Śayitapaścimatāna

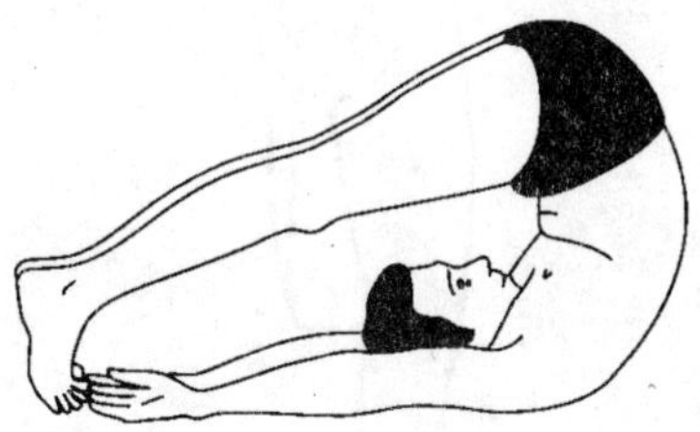

Vicitrakaraṇi

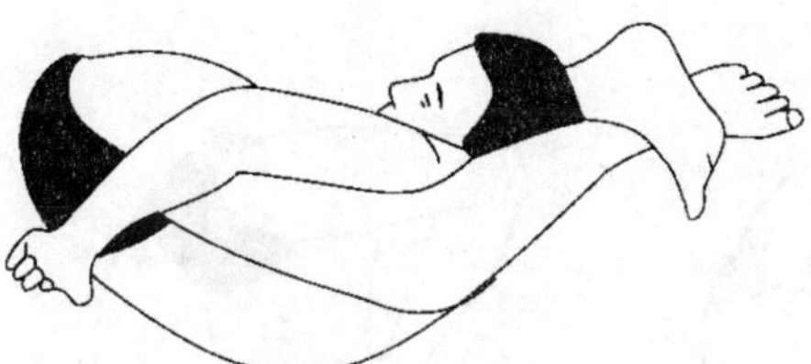

Yoganidrā

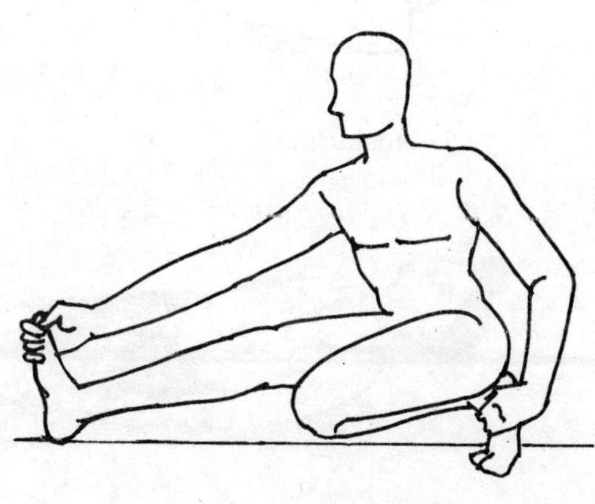

Vidhūnana

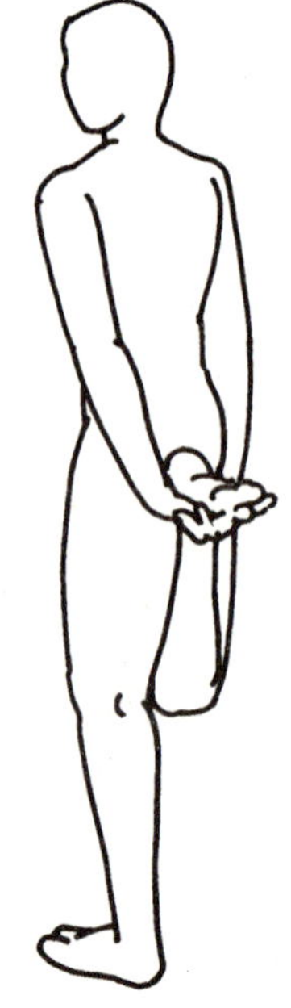

Pādapīḍanāsana

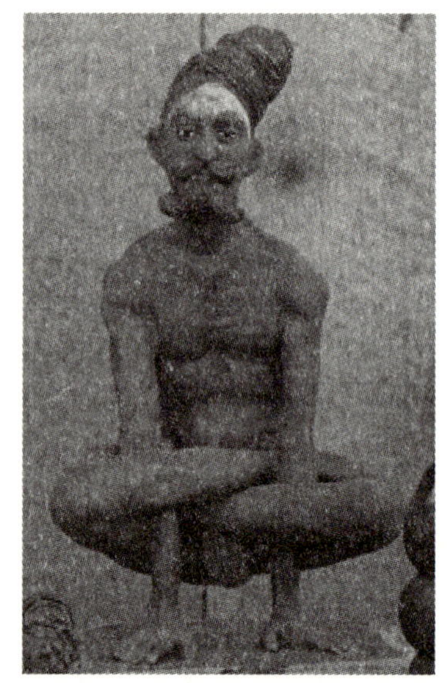

Kukkuṭāsana

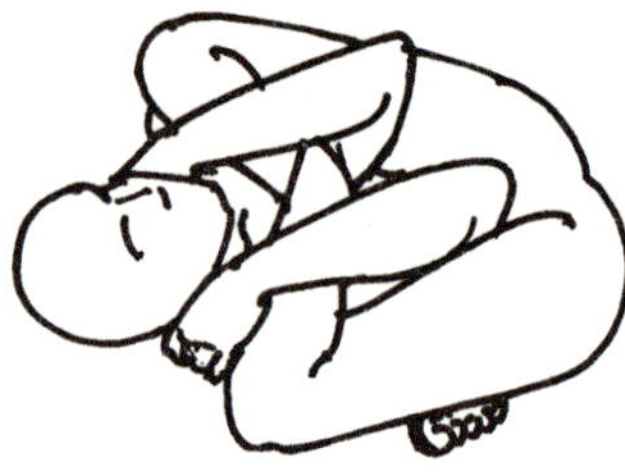

Uttānakūrma

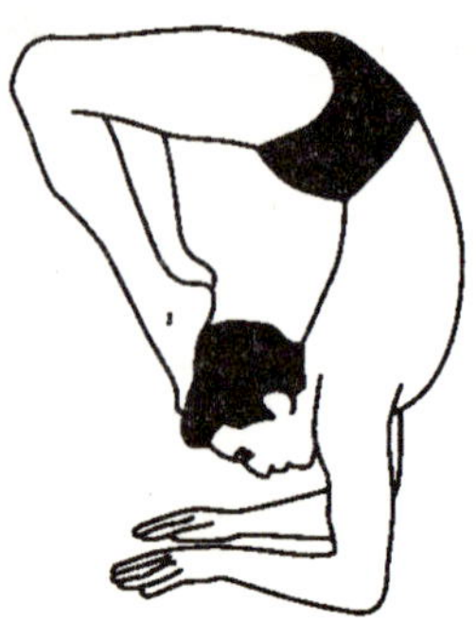

Vṛścikāsana

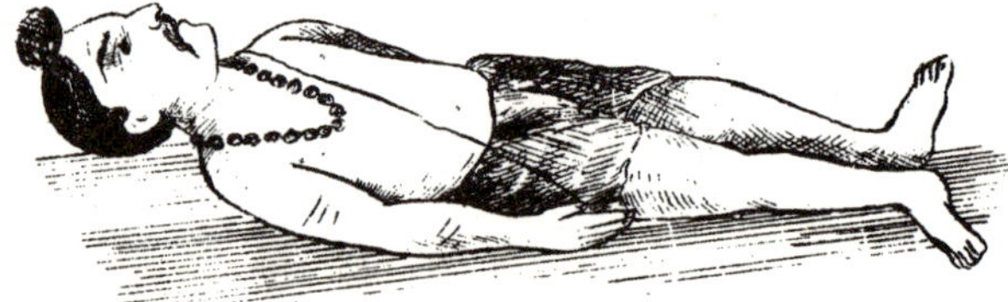

Śavāsana

Appendix-1

[In Tanjavur Ms. No. 6393 (b) the following extra lines appear after this line of verse No. 41 of chapter iv].

"ननु ईश्वरस्यापि पञ्चवक्त्रस्थितपञ्चदृगित्यादिनागमेषु शरीरेन्द्रिययोगः श्रूयते। अत आह पञ्चमन्त्रतनुः। अयमभिप्रायः। ध्यानार्थमेवेश्वरस्य पञ्चवक्त्राद्याकारः श्रूयते। निराकारे ध्यानपूजाद्ययोगात्। यदाहुः। आकारवांस्त्वं नियमादुपास्यो नस्त्वनाकारमुपैति बुद्धिरिति। श्रीमत्पौष्करे साधकस्य तु लक्षार्थं तस्य रूपमिदं स्मृतमिति। अतः पञ्चमन्त्रात्मिकाः पञ्चकृत्योपयोगिन्यः। ईशानाद्याः शुक्तय एव शरीरकार्यं कुर्वाणाः तनुरित्यपचारादुच्यन्ते। यच्छ्रयते। तद्वपुः पञ्चभिर्मन्त्रैः पञ्चकृत्योपयोगिभिः। ईशतत्पुरुषा घोरवामाद्यैर्मस्तकादिकमिति। अत एवाह पञ्चविधं तत्कृत्यं सृष्टिस्थितिसंहृतितिरोभावाः। तद्वदनुग्रहकरणं प्रोक्तम् सततोदितस्यास्य। एतच्च कृत्य पञ्चकं शुद्धा साक्षाच्छिवकर्तृकमशुद्ध्वा ध्वनित्वसंगादि द्वारेन्युक्तम्। श्रीमत्किरणे शुद्धेऽध्वनिः शिवः कर्ता प्रोक्ताऽनन्तो सिते प्रभुरिति। तत्र शिवस्य इष्टिबिन्द्वात्मकादुपादानाच्छुद्धतत्वभुवनाद्युत्पादनपूर्व तदभवनवासिनां विद्यां विद्येश्वराणां च बैन्दव- शरीरयोन्मननादिक्रमेण शब्दोत्पादश्च। अनन्तादि- द्वारासु मायाख्याद्यशुद्धं तत्वाद्युत्पादनपूर्व- पशुसंघानां सूक्ष्मतात्विकशरीरेण स्वकर्मानुगुण- भौवशरीरेण च योजनम्। मन्त्रेश्वराणामधिकारे निबन्धनशरीरोत्पादनस्थितिस्वशक्त्या निरुद्धस्य सर्वस्य जगतः स्वविषय एव स्थानम्। संसृतिः शुद्धा शुद्धाशुद्धकार्यवर्गयोर्बिन्दु मामात्मनो रूपसंहारः। तिरोभावश्च पाशानुग्रहेणात्मना यथागुणभोगभाजनम्। अनुग्रहोऽपि पाशतिरोधानेनाणूनां परापरमोक्षदानमिति। ननु स्थितिसंरक्षणादान् भावानुग्रहकाराश इति। श्रीमद्रौरवातिश्रुते विद्येशानामपि पञ्चकृत्यकारत्वात् कथं स ततोदितस्येति प्राप्तिसाधने दीक्षादिनोपाय- कलापेन प्रतिपदार्थे संग्रहः कथ्यते। अनवश्चात्मन इत्यनेन पशुत्ववियोगिनां विज्ञानाक नां बन्धात्मनां पशुपदार्थत्वमुच्यते। अर्थपञ्चकमित्यनेन मलरोधशक्तिकर्ममायाबिन्दवः प्रोच्यन्ते। ततस्तेषां पञ्चानां बिन्दुमायोद्भूतैः शुद्धाशुद्धरूपैस्तन्व- भुवनभूतभावैः सह पाशपदार्थैः संग्रहः। ननु कथमेकस्याः एव शिवशक्तेः प्रतिपदार्थे च संग्रहं उच्यते परमार्थतः प्रतिपदार्थ एव शक्तेरन्तर्भावः पाशत्वं तु तस्याः पाशधर्मानुवर्तनेनोपचारात्। यदुक्तम् तासां माहेश्वरीशक्तिः

सर्वानुग्राहिका शिवा। धर्मानुवर्तना इत्यपचार्य इति। अस्तु तर्हि मुक्तात्मनां पाशसंसर्गरहितत्वात् शिवत्वम्। विश्वेश्वरादीनाम् बैन्दवशरीरयोगेऽपि कथं पशुत्वापगमः। मुक्तात्मनोऽपि शिवा मुक्तात्मानं सम्प्राप्य शिवसाम्याः। अपि शब्दाद्विश्वेश्वरादयश्च शिवा एव पशुत्वाख्येन मलेन विरहात्। तद्योगिनां हि पशुत्वं पशुसंयोगादिति श्रुतिः। अत एषां शिवत्वेन सर्वज्ञत्वादिना योगाच्छिवत्वमेवम्। बैन्दवादिशरीरयोगस्त्वधिकारमलांशातशेषतोऽधिकार- निबन्धन एव। अतएव च मायोत्रीर्नत्वान्मलरहितत्वाच्च विद्या विश्वेश्वर– पदप्राप्ते परमुक्तित्वम्। कथं पुनर्मन्त्रेश्वराणां कलादियोगात् मलरहितत्वात् कलादीनां योगस्य मायागर्भा धिकारत्वे बन्धनत्वेन तेषामवश्यत्वाच्च। यदुक्तं कालयोगेऽपि नो वश्याः कलानां पशुसंघवदिति। यद्येवं शिवत्वे समाने मुक्तात्मादिभ्योऽस्य परमे। किन्त्वेते प्रसादतः मुक्ताः सोऽनादिमुक्त एको विज्ञेय अनादिमुक्तस्वभाव–सिद्धनित्यानिर्म लनिरतिशय सर्वार्थः ॥"

ଓଃଓ

Variations in the names of *siddhas* mentioned in the *Haṭharatnāvalī* and *Haṭhapradīpikā*

Nos	*Haṭharatnāvalī* (Lonavla Yoga Institute Ed.)	*Haṭhapradīpikā* (Kaivalyadhama Ed. (Hp-Kdm)	*Haṭhapradīpikā* (10 chapters-Lonavla Yoga Institute Ed.)	Variant readings from foot-notes of these books	
1	*Śrīādinātha*	*Śrīādinātha*	*Ādinātha*		
2	*Matsyendra*	*Matsyendra*	*Matsyendra*		
3	*Śābara*	*Śābara*	*Śārada*	*Śāradā* (HP,Kdm)	*Śāradā* (HP, 10ch)
4	*Ānandabhairava*	*Ānandabhairava*	*Ānandabhairava*		
5	*Śāraṅgī*	*Cauraṅgī*	*Cauraṅgī*		
6	*Mīna*	*Mīna*	*Mīna*		
7	*Gorakṣa*	*Gorakṣa*	*Gorakṣa*		
8	*Virūpākṣa*	*Virūpākṣa*	*Virūpākṣa*		
9	*Bileśaya*	*Bileśaya*	*Bileśaya*		
10	*Manthānabhairava*	*Manthānabhairava*	*Manthānabhairava*		
11	*Siddhabuddhi*	*Siddhi* (ii.1) *Buddhi* (ii.11)	*Siddhabuddhi*	*Siddhibuddhi*-HR	*Siddhabuddha* (HP-Kdm)
12	*Kandalī*	*Kanthaḍī*	*Kanthaḍī*		*Kadalā* (HP-Kdm)
13	*Korandaka*	*Koraṇṭaka*	*Kauraṇṭaka*	*Gonandaka*-HR	*Pauraṇthaka,Ghor-aṇṭaka* (HP-Kdm)
14	*Surānanda*	*Surānanda*	*Surānanda*		
15	*Siddhipāda*	*Siddhipāda*	*Siddhapāda*		
16	*Carpaṭi*	*Carpaṭi*	*Carpaṭi*	*Parpaṭi*-HR	*Sarpati* (HP-Kdm)
17	*Karoṭi*	*Kānerī*	*Kānerī*		*Kāvārī, karaṇī* (HP-Kdm)

Nos	***Haṭharatnāvalī*** **(Lonavla Yoga Institute Ed.)**	***Haṭhapradīpikā*** **(Kaivalyadhama Ed. (Hp-Kdm)**	***Haṭhapradīpikā*** **(10 chapters-Lonavla Yoga Institute Ed.)**	**Variant readings from foot-notes of these books**	
18	*Pūjyapāda*	*Pūjyapāda*	*Siddhipāda*		
19	*Nityanātha*	*Nityanātha*	*Nityanātha*		*Bilvanātha, Dhvaninātha* (HP-Kdm)
20	*Nirañjana*	*Nirañjana*	*Nirañjana*		
21	*Kapālī*	*Kapālī*	*Kapālī*		*Kāpālī* (HP-Kdm)
22	*Bindunātha*	*Bindunātha*	*Bindunātha*		
23	*Kākacaṇḍīśvara*	*Kākacaṇḍīśvara*	*Kākacaṇḍīśvara*	*Kākacaṇḍaścaromakaḥ*	*Kākacaṇḍīkharādi* (HP-Kdm)
24	*Allama*	*Allāma*	*Allamāprabhudeva*		*Āllamaprabhu* (HP-Kdm)
25	*Prabhudeva*	*Prabhudeva*			
26	*Naiṭacūṭi*	*Ghoḍācolī*	*Ghorācolī*	*Phaiṭichoṭi* (HR)	*Ghoḍācūlī, Pogavālī* (HP-Kdm)
27	*ṭinṭini*	*ṭinṭinī*	*ṭinṭini*		*ṭhinṭhini* (HP-Kdm)
28	*Bhāluki*	*Bhānukī*	*Vāsukī*	*Tāluki* (HR)	*Bāluki, Tālukī, Mallakī* (HP-Kdm)
29	*Nāgabodha*	*Nāradeva*	*Nāgabodha*	*Nāgalodha* (HR)	*Namideva, Nāgadeva* (HP-Kdm)
30	*Khanḍakāpālika*	*Khanḍa*	*Khanḍa*	*Kanḍī* (HP-10ch)	
31		*Kāpālika*	*Kāpālika*		

Appendix—3

(Some of the āsanas mentioned in the list but not described in the text are described here from other sources.)

Kārmukāsana—Following technique is described in the *Yogāsanam*: "Sit in a cross-legged position. Hold the right big toe with the right hand and left big toe with the left hand and sit erect."

Haṃsāsana— *Kiraṇabhāṣya* of *Śrīkṛṣṇa-vallabhācārya* on PYS (i.46) describes this *āsana* as follows: "Place the two palms on the ground, bring the elbows together and rest the navel region of the abdomen on the elbows. Stretch the legs on the ground and remain steady."

However, *Kapālakuraṇṭaka* gives a different technique. "Assuming *kukkuṭāsana* raise the thighs upto the shoulders. This is *haṃsāsana*".

Cakrāsana—*Kiraṇabhāṣya* of *Śrīkṛṣṇa-vallabhācārya* on PYS (ii.46) describes *cakrāsana* as follows: "Hold the toes of the two feet with the fingers of respective hands. With this position lie on the back imitating the moving wheel."

Yogasiddhāntacandrikā gives a little different technique: "In *śavāsana* the two legs should be taken quickly behind the head and are crossed."

Ahirbudhnyasaṃhitā (31033) and *Varāhopaniṣad* (v.17) describe *cakrāsana* as a meditative posture. They give the technique as follows: "Place the left thigh on the right ankle and the right thigh on the left ankle and keep the trunk erect."

Kūrmāsana— *Haṭhapradīpikā* describes the *kūrmāsana* as follows: "Pressing the anus well with the two ankles, feet everted, one should sit in a calm and composed manner."

Triśikhibrāhmaṇopaniṣad (38) gives the same technique but under the name of *yogāsana*.

Citrapīṭha—*Jogapradīpakā* of *Jayatarāma* and *Yogāsanamālā* describe this *āsana* as below: "Bring the two soles together. With the help of the left elbow raise both the feet over the head and hold them there. With the right hand hold the neck on the left and bring its elbow upto the navel and abdomen. Direct the gaze at the nose."

Gorakṣāsana—*Gheraṇḍasaṃhitā* (ii.24-25) describes this *āsana* as follows: "Keeping the two feet turned upwards between the knees and the thighs, hiding the ankles with upturned hands and contracting the throat, one should gaze at the tip of the nose."

Aṅguṣṭhāsana—*Kiraṇaṭikā* by *Śrīkṛṣṇa-vallabhācārya* on PYS (ii.46) gives the technique as follows: "Sit on the toes and touch the two knees together on the ground. Place the buttocks on the heels and fold the hands on the chest."

Vyāghrāsana—*Kiraṇaṭikā* by *Śrīkṛṣṇa-vallabhācārya* on PYS (ii.46) describes it as follows: "Arrange the legs as in *siṃhāsana*. Place the two hands on the ground by the side of the knees. Bend a little forward, open the mouth, put the tongue out and sit with the eyes dilated."

Śara(la)bhāsana—The text '*Cauryāsī Āsane*' describes this *āsana* as follows: "Lie prone. Place both the palms under the chest. Raise the head up and hold the position."

Gheraṇḍa Saṃhitā (ii.359) describes the technique as follows: "Lie prone pressing the ground with the palms placed on either side of the chest and raise legs together nine inches high in the air. This is called *śalabhāsana* by eminent sages."

Krauñcāsana—The following description of *krauñcāsana* is found in the *Śrītatvanidhi* (67) edited by N. E. Sjoman under the title "The Yoga Tradition of the Mysore Palace". "Open the closed fists between the thighs and knees and take hold of a rope with them. Hold a weight in the teeth and ascend the rope. This is *krauñcāsana*, the crane."

The same description is found also in the *Kapālakuraṇṭaka*.

Dṛḍhāsana—*Kiraṇabhāṣya* of *Śrīkṛṣṇa-vallabhācārya* on PYS (i.46) describes its technique as follows: "Lie on the left side. Bend the left arm in the elbow and support the head with the hand, elbow resting on the ground."

ঙ্গ

Glossary

ādhāracakra —	a synonym for *mūlādhāra.*
advaita —	the one Absolute.
āgama —	a traditional doctrine or precept, a sacred writing or scripture.
ajñāna —	ignorance which conceals wisdom, making people illusioned.
amaravāruṇī —	the divine ambrosia, the secretion from the moon.
akṣara —	a synonym for *māyā* and *prakṛti.*
amarī--	urine, drinking and snuffing of which is recommended while undergoing the course of *vajrolī.* This practice is called *amarolī.*
amarolī —	daily practice of tasting and snuffing of urine which forms a part of *vajrolī* practice.
antaḥkaraṇa —	the internal organs which are *manas, buddhi, citta* and *ahaṅkāra.*
apathya —	food that is contradicted for consumption.
ārambha —	the first of the four states of *yoga.*
avyākṛta —	a synonym for *prakṛti.*
bandha —	the attribute of bondage which is attached to an embodied soul.
bhānu —	a synonym for the sun located at the navel which saps up the nectar flowing from the moon in the head.
bhūta —	the elements which are five, i.e., earth, water, fire, air and ether.
bhūta —	the living creature.
bhūtātmā —	the Cosmic Self which pervades everything.
bimba(dvaya) —	the (pair of) discs of sun and moon.
bindu —	used for *rajas*; also for the centrally aroused light which a *yogī* sees within; generally used for semen; a secretion of the spinal fluid in the *yonisthāna.*
bindujaya —	control of *bindu*—the vital energy of the body.

bindusthairya— stabilization of *bindu.*
brahmacakra— a synonym for *brahmarandhra.*
brahmanāḍī— synonym for *suṣumnā.* Movement of *prāṇa* in this *nāḍī* is highly emphasized as essential for higher achievements in the path of *yoga.*
brahmāṇḍa— the macrocosmic body.

candra— the moon or *iḍā* which is cool in effect. The moon located in the space above the soft palate wherefrom the divine ambrosia oozes.
candramaṇḍala— the moon located at the *kapāla* (forehead).
cāndrī— the divine ambrosia oozing from the *candra* (moon) located in the cavity above the soft palate.
cittavṛttinirodha—control of the modifications of the mind.

dehānala— bodily fire.
dhātu— the bodily constituents which are called *dvīpa* (islands), which are seven in number, i.e., *rasa, rakta, māṃsa, asthi, majjā, śukra* and *medas.*
dhyāna— generally understood as practice of meditation, wherein the mind is made still.

gāyatrī— a Vedic metre of 24 syllables,. The Vedic *mantra* which is as follows—
"*oṃ tat savitur vareṇyaṃ bhargo devasya dhīmahi / dhiyo yo naḥ pracodayāt //*
ghaṭa— the second of the four states of *yoga.*
go— the tongue.
guṇa— the individual quality or qualities of the five elements which are sound, touch, form, taste and smell. The eight supernatural powers like *aṇimā* etc., acquired by an accomplished *yogī.*

hari— the Cosmic soul which pervades everything.

haṭhayoga— the discipline of *yoga* comprises the practice of *ṣaṭkarmas, āsana, kuṃbhaka, mudrā, nādānusandhāna* etc.

iḍā— the left nostril which is of the nature of moon and is *tāmasika* denoting night or inertia. It is also known as *bhāgīrathī.*

indriya— the sense organs.

īśvara— the Supreme Self called *Paramātmā.*

jaṭharāgni— the gastric fire.

jitaśvāsa— one who has mastered the practice of *prāṇāyāma.*

jitendriya— one who has restrained the sense organs.

jīva— the embodied soul attached with *māyā* (illusion).

jīvātman— the embodied soul, the individual Self which has to be freed from the bondage.

jñāna— wisdom.

jñānaśakti— the power of knowledge.

jñānayoga— *yoga* of wisdom, which can sever the relation of attributes attached to an embodied soul.

kaivalya— the Absolute state which arises on dissolution of the mind.

kalā— the tongue which has to be elongated upto the center of the eyebrows by cutting, moving and milking, to attain *khecarī.*

kāladaṇḍa— whip of *kāla*—death or time—that controls all living beings.

kālāgni— fire located at the base *mūlādhāra.*

kālakūṭa— the deadliest of the poisons.

kalpānta— the time of dissolution of the Universe. A *kalpa* is a day of *Brahmā* or 1000 *yugas* being a period of 432 million years of mortals and measuring the duration of the world.

kapāla — the forehead wherein the moon is located.

karaṇa — synonym for *mudrā.*

karma — purificatory process.

kāyasiddhi — attainment of the supernatural bodily powers.

kedāra — the center of the eyebrows which is the confluence of the three rivers, i.e., *nāḍīs— iḍā, piṅgalā* and *suṣumnā.*

kha — the void, wherein the *Ātmā* has to be merged and which has to be perceived everywhere.

kriyāśakti — the three forms of occult power which are *manojavitva* (doing any act any time), *kāmarūpitva* (assuming any form at will) and *vikaraṇabhāva* (infinite mental power to consume and transmit).

kumbhaka — retention of the breath, varieties of *prāṇāyāma* which differ according to *haṭha* texts.

lambikā — the tongue, the practice of cutting, rubbing etc., of the tongue so that it can touch the center of the eyebrows.

laya — it means (i) not to come back to life again, (ii) to forget the objects of experience, (iii) absorption.

layayoga — absorption of the mind in the unstruck sound *(anāhata-nāda).*

mahākhaga — the great bird *prāṇa.*

mahāsiddha — great adepts of *yoga* of the past.

mahāyoga — a synonym for *Pātañjalayoga.*

manaḥsthairya — stability of the mind which is the result of *prāṇāyāma* and which is equated with the state of *manonmanī.*

mantra — a sacred syllable or sentence to be chanted in the prescribed manner.

mantrayoga— *yoga* chiefly comprising chanting of *mantra*.

māruta— *prāṇa* the vital force of life.

maṭha— a hermitage ideal for undertaking *yoga* practices.

maṭhikā— a small cottage which is located in a desolate place where a *yogī* is supposed to reside for *yoga* practices.

māyā— illusion attached to *jīva*—the embodied Self bereft of which, a *jīva* is *sadāśiva* (ever Blissful).

mitāhāra— moderate diet. Consumption of prescribed quality and quantity of food which does not make one feel hungry nor cause drowsiness.

mokṣa— liberation, a state wherein the embodied soul gets freed from all attributes.

mukti— the state of liberation.

nabhojala— the nectar that oozes from the space above the soft palate, onto the fire at the navel causing decay of the human body.

nāda— various sounds heard within the body. The unstruck sound heard within the body, concentration on which results in quick absorption of the mind. It has various levels starting from gross to the subtlest of sounds.

nādānusandhāna—hearing of the unstruck sound *(nāda)* for the absorption of the mind.

nāḍī— conduits in the body through which the vital air *prāṇa* moves. These are considered 72,000 in number.

nāḍīcakra— a *cakra* located at the *mulādhāra* wherefrom the *nāḍīs* originate. It resembles an egg of a hen. The network of the *nāḍīs*. Its purification has been greatly emphasized in *haṭhayoga*.

nāḍīśuddhi — purification of the *nāḍīs* in the body which is judged by the external signs like slimness and luster of the body etc.

nirālamba — a synonym for *Brahma.*

nirañjana — one that is without blemish. A synonym for *Brahma.*

niśā — used as a *kumbhaka*

niṣpatti — the last of the four states of *yoga* which a *yogī* experiences.

paramāṇu — the atoms which come together to form the Universe.

paramātman — the Universal or Cosmic Soul which is ever free.

paricaya — the third of the four states of *yoga* experienced by a *yogī.*

paścimapatha — the posterior path. The *suṣumnā nāḍī.* Moving of *prāṇa* in this *nāḍī* merges the *prāṇa* into the state of *laya* (absorption of the mind) and one overcomes diseases and premature death.

pātāla — the void at the base of the spine wherein consciousness is located.

pathya — recommended food.

piṇḍa — the human body. The microcosmic (individual) body.

piṅgalā — the right nostril which is of the nature of sun and is *rājasika* denoting agility. It is also known as *yamunā.*

pīṭha — a synonym for *āsana.*

pradhāna — the primordial state of *prakṛti*, a synonym for *māyā* or *avyakta.*

praṇava — the sacred syllable *OM.*

prapañca — the perceptible world made out of the *paramāṇus* (atoms).

pratyāhāra — withdrawal of the sense from the sense object.

pṛthvī — the term used for *āsana.*

purāṇa— a legendary history, certain wellknown sacred works which are 18 in number, supposed to have been composed by *Vyāsa* and contain the whole body of Hindu mythology.

puruṣa— the superior Self called *Paramātmā.*

rājadanta— the front teeth.

rajas— one of the triad of *guṇas* standing for activity. Menstrual discharge.

rājayoga— a synonym for *Pātañjalayoga* comprising eight *aṅgas* or components for practice.

śabdagarbhā— tongue, movement of which in a prescribed manner plays a significant role in arousal of *kuṇḍalinī.*

sadāśiva— the Self which is bereft of all attributes.

śakti— a synonym for *kuṇḍalinī* which has to be awakened from its latent and coiled position.

samādhi— Ultimate state of *yogic* endeavour. End of mental construction.

śāṃbhavī— a *mudrā* in which one gazes in between the eyebrows and concentrates his mind inside.

śambhu— an epithet of *Śiva.*

saṅketa— a special apparatus which is shaped like a snake, rounded, having two *śṛṅkhalās* which provides rest for elbow, measuring 72 digits, possession of which is integral for attainment of *khecarī.* Special secret instructions given by a *guru* which have to be incorporated while doing the practice of *āsana, mudrā* etc.

sarasvatī— a synonym for *kuṇḍalinī.*

śaśī— the moon wherefrom the divine nectar flows.

ṣaṭcakra— the six *cakras* or plexuses — *ādhāra, svādhiṣṭhāna, maṇipūra, anāhata, viśuddha* and *ājñā.*

satva— one of the triad of *guṇas* denoting illumination.

siddha— one who has attained success in *yoga.*

siddhipada— the course of *yoga.*

śirājāla— the network of the nerves tying up of which restricts the downward flow of the nectar oozing from the space.

śiras— a Vedic *mantra* attached to the end of the popular *Gāyatrī mantra* which is— *'om āpo jyoti raso'mṛtaṃ brahma bhūr bhuvaḥ svarom'.*

śruti— a sacred Vedic text, the scripture that has been transferred through oral communication.

sūrya— the right nostril or *piṅgalā.* The sun located at the navel which consumes the divine nectar flowing from the moon situated above the soft palate.

suṣira— an aperture located at the base of the spine which is the fountain head of the Consciousness.

suṣupti— one of the four states of Consciousness.

tamas— One of the triad of the *guṇas* representing the quality of inertia.

tatva— basic elements which are twenty four according to *Sāṃkhya*, thirty according to *Paurāṇikas* and thirty six as per the experts of *Śaivāgama.* The Self.

tatvajñāna— knowledge of the Self.

tridaśa— the deities like *Brahmā* etc.

triguṇa— the triad of *guṇas*, namely, *satva, rajas* and *tamas*, which is the cause of the Universe and which holds the key to creation, sustenance and dissolution.

triveṇīsaṅgama— the confluence of the three rivers, i.e. *nāḍīs—iḍā, piṅgalā* and *suṣumnā* at the center of the eyebrows which is called *kedāra*.

unmanībhāva— state of *yoga* wherein the mental fluctuation is completely stopped by moving the *prāṇa* through *suṣumnā.*

vahnimaṇḍala— the navel region wherein the gastric fire is based.

vajrakandara— the urethra.

viṣaya— the objects (of senses).

vyāhṛti— a mystic word from the *Vedas.* They are seven in number like—*bhūḥ, bhuvaḥ, svaḥ, mahaḥ, janaḥ, tapaḥ* and *satyaṃ.*

yogamaṭha— an ideal cottage used by a *yogī* for undertaking *yoga* practices.

yogasiddhi— success in *yoga* which is attained through knowledge of the scriptures, grace of the *guru*, practice of *yoga* and grace of *Īśvara.*

yoginīcakra— powers of the deities presiding over the *cakras.* Important nerve plexus.

yonisthāna— the perineum, the place between the genital and anus wherein coiled *kuṇḍalī* is supposed to be lying latent.

Index of Half-verses

Word Index

(Numbers stand for page numbers).

A

L

M

N

W

Y

The Lonavla Yoga Institute (India)

(Regd. No. 1439/1998/Pune)
B-17, Rachana Gardens, Bhangarwadi
Lonavla-410 401, Pune (India)
Tel: 0091-02114-279333
E-mail: lonayogalnl@vsnl.net
www.lonavalayoga.org

The Lonavla Yoga Institute (India) was founded in May 1996 by **Dr. M. L. Gharote** who was a student and collaborator of **Swami Kuvalayananda**, Founder of Kaivalyadhama Yoga Institute and a Pioneer of Scientific Yoga.

Activities of The Lonavla Yoga Institute (India)

1. To conduct or help conducting research in the field of pure and applied Yoga.
2. To edit or get edited text books on Yoga with notes and translations and publish them.
3. To prepare and publish catalogues, digests, indices or glossaries of Yogic texts and subjects allied to Yoga with a view to help critical studies of Yogic texts.
4. To publish Newsletter "Yoga Pradipa".
5. To organize seminars and conduct courses in Yoga and provide facilities for training individuals or groups of individuals in India or abroad.
6. To establish contacts and co-operate with the individuals and associations or organizations working in the field of Yoga in different aspects.
7. To give adequate guidance to the individuals and groups in the Yogic therapeutic matters.

Projects at hand

i. Publication of Yoga texts with translations in different languages.
ii. Catalogue of Yoga Manuscripts.
iii. Organization of Yoga Therapy Courses in different places with the help of affiliated or related Associations and Institutions.
iv. Organization of Yoga workshops.

Publications

Within a short period of its existence the Institute has published the following books:

1. **Glossary of Yoga Texts** — Dr. M. L. Gharote.
2. **Swami Kuvalayananda — A Pioneer of Scientific Yoga and Physical Education** —
   Dr. M. L. Gharote and Dr. Manmath M. Gharote.
3. **Yogic Techniques**— Dr. M. L. Gharote.
4. **Hatha Pradipika Vrtti by Bhojatmaja (Marathi)** —
   Ed. Dr. M. L. Gharote.
5. **Kumbhaka Paddhati or Science of Pranayama** —
   Ed. Dr. M. L. Gharote & Parimal Devnath.
6. **Hathapradipika (10 chapters) with the Commentary — Yogaprakasika by Balakrishna** —Second Revised Edition
   Ed. Dr. M. L. Gharote & Parimal Devnath.
7. **Yuktabhavadeva of Bhavadeva Mishra** (Original Sanskrit Text, English Summary and Critical Appraisal) —
   Ed. Dr. M. L. Gharote & Dr. V. K. Jha.
8. **An Introduction to Yuktabhavadeva of Bhavadeva Mishra** (English Summary and Critical Appraisal) —
   Ed. Dr. M. L. Gharote & Dr. V. K. Jha.
9. **Hatharatnavali by Srinivasa** — Critical edition, transliteration, translation, figures, notes and appendices. — Ed. Dr. M. L. Gharote
10. **Pranayama- The Science of Breath** — Dr. M. L. Gharote.
11. **Siddhasiddhantapaddhati** — Ed. Dr. M. L. Gharote.
12. **Encyclopaedia of Traditional Asanas** —
    Ed. Dr. M. L. Gharote, Dr. V. K. Jha,
    Dr. Parimal Devnath, Dr. S. B. Sakhalkar.
13. **Hathatattvakaumudi of Sundaradeva** —
    Ed. Dr. M. L. Gharote, Dr. Parimal Devnath r
    Dr. Vijay Kant Jha.
14. **Guidelines for Yogic Practices** — Dr. M. L. Gharote.
15. **Evolution in Yoga** — Dr. Manmath M. Gharote,
    Dr. Parimal Devnath, Dr. V. K. Jha.
16. **Critical Edition of three Selected Yogopanishads** —
    Dr. Manmath M. Gharote, Dr. Parimal Devnath,
    Dr. V. K. Jha.
17. **Yogika Prakriya (Marathi)** — Dr. M. L. Gharote.
18. **Yogika prakriyanche Margadarshan** —
    Dr. M. L. Gharote.

19. **Therapeutic References in Traditional Yoga Texts** — Ed. Dr. Manmath M. Gharote, Dr. V. K. Jha, Dr. Parimal Devnath.

20. **Amanaskayoga** — Dr. Manmath M. Gharote, Dr. V. K. Jha, Dr. Parimal Devnath.

21. **Pranayama - Shwasache Shastra** — Ed. Dr. M. L. Gharote

22. **Maṇḍalabrāhmaṇopaniṣad and Nādabindūpaniṣad** — Dr. Manmath M. Gharote, Dr. Parimal Devnath, Dr. V. K. Jha.

23. **Amṛtavākyam (Hindi)** — Dr. Manmath M. Gharote, Dr. V. K. Jha

24. **Amṛtavākyam (English)** — Dr. Manmath M. Gharote, Dr. V. K. Jha

25. **Dattātreyayogaśāstram** — Dr. Manmath M. Gharote, Dr. Parimal Devnath

<u>Future Publications</u>

The Institute is working on the following texts and soon these will be published.

i. **Critical Editions of Selected Yogopanishads.**

ii. **Natha Vakya.**

iii. **Critical edition of Goraksha Shataka.**

iv. **Concordance of Asanas and Pranayama.**

v. **Akulagama Tantra.**

vi. **Yogic Anatomy and Physiology.**

vii. **Yogabija**

viii. **Notices of Manuscripts on Hathayoga.**

***